A HANDBOOK FOR MEDICAL TEACHERS
Second Edition

A HANDBOOK FOR MEDICAL TEACHERS
Second Edition

DAVID NEWBLE, BSc(Hons), MBChB, MD,
FRACP, DipEd
Reader in Medicine
The University of Adelaide
South Australia

ROBERT CANNON, MA(Hons), MEdAdmin,
DipTertEd
Director
Advisory Centre for University Education
The University of Adelaide
South Australia

Illustrations by **Zig Kapelis,** MArch,
FRAIA
Senior Lecturer in Architecture
The University of Adelaide
South Australia

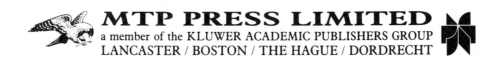
MTP PRESS LIMITED
a member of the KLUWER ACADEMIC PUBLISHERS GROUP
LANCASTER / BOSTON / THE HAGUE / DORDRECHT

Published in the UK and Europe by
MTP Press Limited
Falcon House
Lancaster, England

British Library Cataloguing in Publication Data

Newble, David
    A handbook for medical teachers. -2nd ed.
    1. Medicine–Study and teaching
    I. Title   II. Cannon, Robert   III. Newble,
    David. Handbook for clinical teachers
    610'.7'11   R834

ISBN 0–85200–673–X

Published in the USA by
MTP Press
A division of Kluwer Academic Publishers
101 Philip Drive
Norwell, MA 02061, USA.

Library of Congress Cataloging-in-Publication Data

Newble, David.
    A handbook for medical teachers.

    Rev. ed. of: A handbook for clinical teachers.
1983
    Includes bibliographies and index.
    1. Medicine, Clinical—Study and teaching—
Handbooks, manuals, etc. 2. Medicine—Study and
teaching—Handbooks, manuals etc. I. Cannon,
Robert (Robert Anthony) II. Newble, David.
A handbook for clinical teachers. III. Title.
[DNLM: 1. Education Medical—handbooks. 2. Teaching—
methods—handbooks. W. 39 N534h]
R834.N49   1987   610.7'11   87–4081
ISBN 0–85200–673–X

Printed by Butler and Tanner Ltd, Frome and London

CONTENTS

FOREWORD

More than thirty years ago I began my studies of medical education in the United States. At that time I was an associate professor of education and totally unfamiliar with medical education. Indeed, when I was asked whether I though someone with expertise in education might be helpful to medical educators, my response was simple, direct and to the point: "I have never set foot inside a medical school and therefore do not know anything about medical education." What began for me then was an intensive orientation to American medical education: observation of all kinds of teaching; interviews with faculty and students; participation in committee meetings, conferences, and rounds; and discussion of all of these experiences with medical school teachers and administrators.

Six months later my understanding of the medical education world had reached a stage at which I thought I might be helpful to some teachers with regard to certain problems. One of the major findings of my six months of immersion in American medical education was that teachers were not prepared for their roles as teachers. Some of them were excellent teachers; some of them were not very good teachers; some of them wanted to understand the teaching–learning process; some of them did not want to learn about teaching and learning.

Today, thirty years later, medical educators are far better off in that there are resources available to teachers to help them become better teachers: courses, workshops, seminars, fellowships. Moreover, the research efforts in medical education and the development of newer approaches have provided dramatic impetus for the improvement of teaching in medical schools. And the pioneering activities of a few have lead to the involvement of many in seeking new – and better – ways. Furthermore, from the workshops, seminars and courses, materials have been produced and tested in the very setting in which they are to be used.

The medical school teacher of today who wants to learn something about medical education, who wants to improve his or her teaching practices, who wants to explore other approaches to helping students learn, now can rely on the accumulated results of these decades of resesarch and development dedicated specifically to **medical** education. For the novice medical school teacher, both principles and practices can be learned from readily available materials.

The most promising of these developments over the years seem always to have been the result of collaborative efforts of those with expertize in education and those with familiarity with medicine and medical education. Indeed, the original efforts of George Miller, Stephen Abrahamson, Edwin Rosinski and the rest of a pioneering group in the Project in Medical Education at the University of Buffalo involved that collaborative model for all the years of that Project. That 'model' produced remarkable results, chronicled in Miller's *Educating Medical Teachers*, and the most successful continuing efforts have been those involving collaboration of those from medicine (who have learned something about education) and those from education (who have learned something about medical education).

Textbooks of pedagogy are surely not new! But books designed to help teachers in professional schools (e.g. medical schools, dental schools, nursing schools) did not exist at the time when we first became involved in medical education. Some 'educationists' suggested that the available books in general pedagogy could surely serve that purpose. Saner heads prevailed, however, and over the years, slowly but surely, materials have been developed – materials that include basic educational principles along with realistic, practical applications and illustrations all drawn from medical education. *A Handbook for Medical Teachers* offers exactly what I have been talking about: a useful guidebook which includes relevant illustrations from the world of medical education, all based on sound educational principles. Imagine the contribution to a new teacher in a school of medicine: an opportunity to learn something about educational processes and practices in the context of theory and principles – and all in a non-threatening, indeed rather attractive manner.

But my purpose in this Foreword should not be to 'sell' the book; it really is to muse about progress in medical education and marvel at the swiftness and slowness of that progress. We still find medical school teachers who have no wish to learn anything about education; we still find medical school teachers who denigrate efforts at improvement of teaching practices; we still find that medical school teachers begin a career in medical education with no specific preparation for their roles as teachers. That's the 'slowness'. But now we have materials for those who want to learn about education. And the materials are specific to the needs of the medical school teachers. That's the 'swiftness'.

The recent publication of **Physicians for the Twenty-First Century**, the report of the Panel on the General Professional Education of the Physician (the GPEP Report of the Association of American Medical Colleges), has dramatically stimulated American medical educators to a thoughtful review of medical education. It includes a most relevant recommendation: "Medical schools should establish programs to assist members of the faculty to expand their teaching capabilities beyond their specialized fields to encompass as much of the full range of ... education of students as is possible." Such an acknowledgement in that document could serve alone as a Foreword to this book. The need is still with us after all these years. The difference is that now we have the tools to do the job.

Stephen Abrahamson, PhD,
Professor and Chairman,
Department of Medical Education,
University of Southern California,
Los Angeles
USA

PREFACE TO SECOND EDITION

The need for a handbook on teaching has clearly been established by the positive response we have received to the first edition. This response has been reflected in the need for several reprintings and sales of foreign printing rights. It has also come from published reviews and informal feedback from readers in many parts of the world. We have been gratified to find that the book has been found to be useful by teachers outside medical schools. These have not only included dentists, nurses and allied health professionals, but also teachers outside the medical arena.

An unexpected bonus for us has been the requests we have received to conduct workshops and courses, both in Australia and overseas. We have found the Handbook to be an excellent course-book and priced at a level which allows it to be included in registration costs. We have discovered others using it for the same purpose and it may be an idea that more of our educational colleagues would wish to consider.

As one constant criticism has been of the title, being thought to inadequately reflect the breadth of the contents, we have decided to rename the second edition **A Handbook for Medical Teachers**. We hope this will be taken to include medical teachers in the widest sense and will encourage its use by those not directly involved in clinical teaching. The messages are, we believe, equally relevant to all teachers.

In approaching the revision of the book, we were concerned to discover how well we were meeting the needs of the target audience – the average busy medical teacher. We therefore conducted a questionnaire survey of a sample of those who had purchased the book and who were working in a variety of different teaching situations within and outside medical institutions. All responses were very favourable, but some provided us with suggestions for alterations and additions. One common suggestion was to provide more advice on what to do when things go wrong and this we have attempted to do. We have also set out to introduce some of the newer educational ideas that have become prevalent over the last five years.

One new chapter has been included entitled 'Helping Students Learn'. Though we hope that each chapter in the book is relevant to such an aim, the focus is very much on helping the teacher perform a variety of tasks more effectively. We believe it is also necessary for teachers to be more mindful of the problems some students have with their studies and to have some basis on which to recognize them and provide assistance.

We look forward to receiving as much feedback about this edition as we did from the first.

Finally, we would like to express appreciation to our secretarial staff and particularly to Chris Timms and Phil Johnstone of MTP Press for their continued support and enthusiasm.

David Newble
Robert Cannon
Adelaide, 1987

PREFACE TO FIRST EDITION

Medical students are to a large extent taught by people who have undertaken little or no formal study in the field of education. Although formal study of any subject is no guarantee of satisfactory on-the-job performance, teaching practice itself without a knowledge of the fundamental principles of education is likely to bring distortions into the teaching situation. Our own experience leads us to believe that many teachers are concerned at this lack of expertise. This concern is manifest by their willing participation in activities which provide them with practical assistance in improving their educational skills. Unfortunately, few books have been written to aid the average clinical teacher wishing to gain a perspective on basic educational principles or seeking suggestions on how these might be applied to teaching.

A previous publication by the Advisory Centre for University Education (ACUE) at the University of Adelaide, entitled *University Teaching*, has proved to be very popular, both locally and overseas, and has clearly met the needs of organizers and participants in teacher training programmes in tertiary institutions. The success of this publication, and our experience with a variety of educational activities organized for staff of medical and dental schools and postgraduate organizations, led us to believe that a pragmatic educational guide for medical teachers would be of value to all such teachers and particularly to those asked to undertake an educational task for the first time.

We wish to make it clear that this book is not a comprehensive textbook of education and neither is it designed to be read from cover to cover, though we have no objection to anyone doing so if they wish. Rather, our aim has been to provide a resource for the busy teacher faced with undertaking the educational tasks which must inevitably come his way, and wishing to approach such tasks with a confidence based on reliable information. We are mindful that no doctor would consider instituting treatment on a patient having a condition with which he was not familiar without at least reading about such treatment in a reliable book or article. Likewise, it is reasonable to expect a teacher to approach a teaching task with a similar degree of responsibility. We would therefore expect the teacher to use the book selectively based on need.

As one of the authors is a physician, the perspective of the book is that of medical education. Consequently most of the examples have a clinical flavour. This has been done deliberately in order to guarantee that we only make recommendations and give illustrations based on our own experience and which we know to have been successful. However, we have no reason to believe that this book will not be of equal interest and value to all tertiary teachers and particularly to those concerned with professional education at undergraduate and postgraduate level. This belief is supported by positive comments from a variety of our colleagues in different faculties who have seen copies of the manuscript.

Perhaps we should add a word about our layout and illustrations. Too many books, we fear, are needlessly unattractive because of their presentation. Accordingly, many books are not used to their best advantage. It is our hope that the layout and illustrations in this book will not only create interest but also help in the process of learning and application. For his illustrative work and suggestions, we are indebted to Zig Kapelis.

We would like to pay tribute to Professor Stephen Abrahamson, one of the doyens of medical education and the person primarily responsible for stimulating an interest and providing training in education for one of the authors (DN). We also wish to thank our secretaries Barbara Moss, Mary Denys and Aileen Philps for their willing help during the preparation of this book.

David Newble
Robert Cannon
Adelaide, 1983

1: GIVING A LECTURE

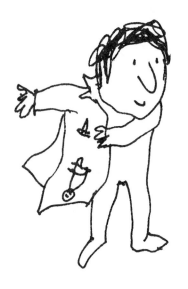

INTRODUCTION

This chapter assumes that you have been asked to give a lecture or series of lectures and that you are keen to enhance the chances of the students learning and remembering what you have taught. To do this you will need a basic understanding of the factors which are likely to influence the learning of the students during the lecture as well as a range of suitable techniques.

STUDENT LEARNING

Educational research allows us to make a few broad generalizations about student learning in a lecture situation. On the basis of current research, Bligh argues persuasively that the lecture is as effective as most other methods of transmitting information but is less effective than other methods for promoting thought or changing attitudes. However, it is still possible to achieve the latter in the lecture hall using techniques discussed later.

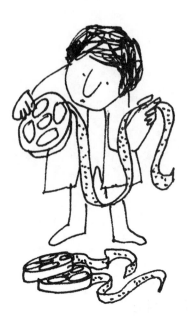

Important considerations in learning are memory, arousal, motivation, structure and feedback. **Memory** has two components – short term and long term. In essence, your task is to get accurate information into short term memory and aid its rapid transfer into long term memory. Only a limited amount of information can be retained in the short term memory and its half life is very brief. It is vulnerable to many outside influences, some of which can be minimized by the lecturer. Information will not be transferred to long term memory unless it is understood. This cannot be achieved unless the student is attending to what you are saying, a state of affairs which will be determined by his level of arousal and degree of motivation. **Arousal** implies a general state of readiness of the brain to accept new information and **motivation** implies a willingness to direct its activity to a specific task. Above all else the teacher's role is to increase the level of arousal and to maintain it. What happens, hypothetically, to a student's level of performance during a traditional uninterrupted lecture is graphically displayed by the heavy line in Figure 1.1. It shows a rapid and continuous decline after the first few minutes with a slight renewal of interest just before the end. The graph also indicates the potential value of a rest period which increases attention and results in a learning gain outweighing the amount of learning lost during the rest period. Interestingly, a graph of lecturer performance would closely parallel that of student performance.

FIGURE 1·1

HYPOTHESIZED PATTERN OF STUDENT LEVEL OF PER- FORMANCE SHOWING A PROGRESSIVE FALL IN ATTENTION AND LEARNING DURING AN UNINTERRUPTED LECTURE AND CONTRASTING THIS WITH THE GAIN OBTAINED FROM INTRODUCING A REST PERIOD (AFTER BLIGH, 1971)

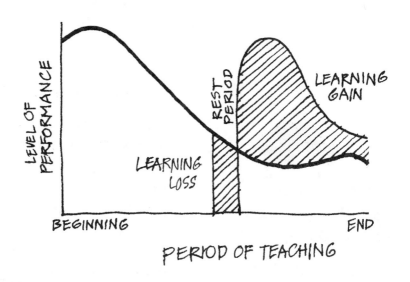

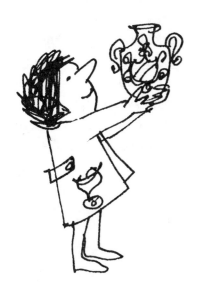

Motivation is such a key factor that it appears to be more important in learning than intelligence. The difficulty is that not all students are motivated by the same thing. Among the more common motivators are the relevance of the material to their ultimate careers, the generation of a feeling of curiosity early in the lecture, the enthusiasm of the teacher for the subject, positive feedback and, not surprisingly, examinations.

Having attained the required degree of arousal and motivation you will still not succeed unless you use a technique which aids the students' understanding of the material to be presented. The lecture must be organized into a **logical structure** which is comprehended by the class. It is appropriate to describe this at the beginning of the lecture or present it in a visual form (blackboard, overhead transparency, handout). You should also be aware that remembering will be further enhanced by giving relevant examples of the points made, by explaining new concepts in terms of familiar ones (i.e. using analogies) and by incorporating opportunities for the students to review and use the information already covered. Specific techniques of doing so are described later.

Feedback, particularly positive feedback in which reward is more prominent than punishment, is a proven adjunct to learning. One study showed that students tested on the subject material at the end of a lecture retained more over the next few weeks than those not tested.

Effectiveness of learning is also enhanced if your lecture supports and builds on previous information. This highlights the need for the lecturer to avoid making rash assumptions about knowledge obtained from previous lectures and courses.

THE PURPOSE OF THE LECTURE

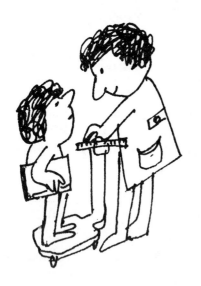

As a rule lecturers attempt to achieve too much in their lectures. This problem is aggravated if the task is to give a single lecture on a specific topic rather than a series of lectures to cover a wider area. In general terms, you should decide whether the main purpose of the lecture is to motivate the students so that they appreciate the importance of the subject material in the overall scheme of things, whether it is to transmit a body of information not readily attainable elsewhere or whether it is to have the student leave the theatre having learned some important concepts and principles. True, you may be forced to try and achieve all of these in a single lecture. If so, it should be structured to deal with them sequentially not concurrently. Trade-offs will then have to be made to allow adequate time for each component. If you are lucky enough to have a series of lectures to give then the problems are not so great.

THE CONTEXT OF THE LECTURE

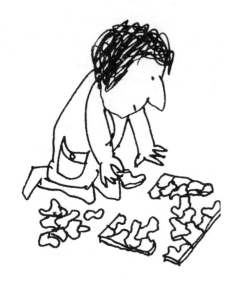

Your lecture has a place in the curriculum and hopefully a carefully planned place. All too frequently, however, the only information you will receive from the planners will be the title of the lecture. As a minimum, you will then need to obtain a copy of the relevant part of the curriculum to see how your subject fits in. You might try contacting the curriculum committee or head of the department for specific details of what they wish you to teach. Do not be surprised if you are told that you are the expert and should know what the students should be taught! You may also try talking to the lecturers preceding you, particularly those whom you might sublimely assume will teach some facts or principles on which you intend to rely. In general it is unwise to assume that the students have learned (even if they have been taught) anything that is vital to their understanding of your lecture. It is only after a realistic appraisal of the context of your contribution that you can rationally set about its planning.

WHAT DO THE STUDENTS REQUIRE OF THE LECTURER?

Several studies have attempted to define what students think are the characteristics of a good lecturer. One such list includes forty-three components, the most frequently quoted of which are seen in Figure 1.2. It would be well worth self-critically evaluating your lecture performance against these criteria.

FIGURE 1.2

SOME ATTRIBUTES OF THE GOOD LECTURER (AFTER COOPER AND FOY, 1967)

- Presents the material clearly and logically.
- Enables the student to understand the basic principles of the subject.
- Can be heard clearly.
- Makes the material intelligibly meaningful.
- Adequately covers the ground.
- Maintains continuity in the course.
- Is constructive and helpful in his criticism.
- Shows an expert knowledge of the subject.
- Adopts an appropriate pace during the lecture.
- Includes material not readily accessible in textbooks.
- Is concise.
- Illustrates the practical applications of the theory of the subject.

PREPARING THE LECTURE

Define the purpose

Having clarified the context of the lecture to the best of your ability the time has come to get down to some detailed planning. The best way to start is to write down the purpose(s) of the lecture. We say write down advisedly because nothing clarifies the mind more than putting pen to paper!

Identify the content

Now set about identifying the content. We suggest you start by initially jotting down the main ideas or theories that come to mind around the central purpose of the lecture. This should be done during a period of free thinking without any particular concern for the order in which you may eventually wish to present them in the lecture. Figure 1.3 illustrates a way of doing this which has been found to be helpful by staff attending our courses for new lecturers.

The lecture topic (in this case, hypertension) is placed in the centre of the paper and the main points to be made are written down as indicated. As the main ideas are identified,

FIGURE 1·3
METHOD OF
IDENTIFYING
THE CONTENT
FOR A LECTURE
(AFTER BUZAN,
1974)

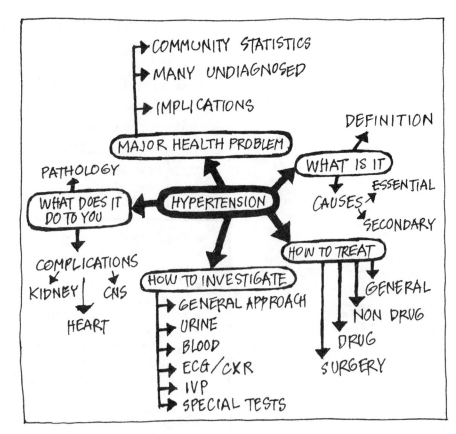

further points will tend to branch out as you think more carefully about them. This process is continued until you have ex-
hausted all your ideas. You may at this stage find that you
need to read around some of the ideas in order to refine them
or to bring yourself up to date.

During this exercise you will find that illustrative examples of
key points come to mind. Jot these down also. In addition you
should be on the look out for illustrations from which you
might prepare slides or other audiovisual aids. If you have the
personality for it, appropriate jokes or cartoons may be
collected.

Finalize the plan

Now you must finalize the plan of the lecture. The rough
content plan must be transformed into a linear structure
which follows a logical sequence. There is no single best way
of doing so but if you are a novice you may prefer a formal
structure from which to work. One such structure is seen in
Figure 1.4.

FIGURE 1.4

A LECTURE PLAN

1 Introduction and overview

    a.   Describe the purpose of the lecture.
    b.   Outline the key areas to be covered.

2 First key point

    a.   Development of ideas.
    b.   Use of examples.
    c.   Restatement of **first key point**.

3 Second key point

    a.   Development of ideas.
    b.   Use of examples.
    c.   Restatement of **first and second points**.

4 Third key point

    a.   Development of ideas.
    b.   Use of examples.
    c.   Restatement of **first, second and third points**.

5 Summary and conclusion

Part of such a plan that was developed for the lecture on hypertension outlined previously is shown in Figure 1.5. The plan also includes notations for the inclusion of visual material such as overhead transparencies and slides.

FIGURE 1.5

PART OF A DETAILED
LECTURE PLAN

TITLE : HYPERTENSION

1 INTRODUCTION
    FIVE KEY POINTS TO BE COVERED (OVERHEAD)
A . THE NATURE AND EXTENT OF THE PROBLEM
B . WHAT IS HYPERTENSION AND ITS CAUSES
C . WHAT DOES IT DO TO YOU
D . INVESTIGATION
E . TREATMENT

2 THE PROBLEM
    A . DBP >90 LEADS TO SIGNIFICANT MORBIDITY /
        MORTALITY (SLIDE - ACTUAL STATISTICS)
    B . 10-25% ADULT POPULATION HAS HYPERTENSION
        BUT OFTEN UNDIAGNOSED OR INEFFECTIVELY TREATED
    C . TREATMENT REDUCES MORBIDITY / MORTALITY
        (SLIDE - VETERAN'S STUDY FROM USA)
    D . IMPLICATIONS OF SCREENING - DIAGNOSIS, COST,
        EDUCATION

3 WHAT IS HYPERTENSION

    A . MULTIFACTORIAL (SLIDE - VARIOUS FACTORS)
    B . ESSENTIAL AND SECONDARY
    C . CAUSES OF SECONDARY HYPERTENSION
        (SLIDE) .

This is the classical content orientated lecture plan. You may wish to be more ambitious and use a **problem-centred plan**. This requires extra thought but done well is likely to be rewarding. It is a technique suited to the lecture in which the purpose is to get students to learn major concepts and principles rather than to primarily transmit factual information. In this case the lecturer opens with the statement of the problem, often presented in the form of a real-life clinical situation or case history. Students are led through a consideration of a variety of possible solutions. The method is an ideal one for introducing student participation during the lecture.

PRESENTING THE LECTURE

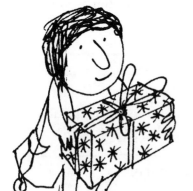

Having decided what you intend to teach you must now give careful attention to how you are going to get it across to the students. Let us assume that it is to be your first contact with this group of students. Your recently acquired knowledge of educational research tells you that before any learning can take place the students must be aroused and you must structure your lecture so that this arousal level is maintained. You may wish to obtain their attention initially by devising an arresting opening to the lecture. Ways of doing this are limited only by your personality and your imagination. A joke, a movie clip, an anecdote, a patient or a discussion with a few of the audience may generate interest. However, it must be born in mind that the attention of the students ought to be engaged by the subject of the lecture and not by the personality of the lecturer. The danger of the latter has become known as the 'Dr Fox effect' based on an experiment where an actor (Dr Fox) gave a lecture comprising meaningless double-talk which fooled experienced listeners into believing that they had participated in a worthwhile and stimulating learning experience.

Starting the lecture

Particular attention needs to be given to the way you start your lecture. For many teachers this is the most difficult aspect of teaching. It is important to decide beforehand exactly how you intend to start. Do not leave this decision until you are facing the students.

Perhaps the easiest way is to explain the purpose of the lecture and how it is organized. An overhead transparency showing an outline of your lecture plan is a good way of doing this. Such visual material will take attention away from yourself, give you something to talk to and allow you to get into your stride.

Once you become a bit more confident other issues should be considered. You must become sensitive to the students' degree of arousal and their motivation to learn your material. It is often helpful to arrive early and chat with some of the students before the lecture to establish their level of previous knowledge. Alternatively, you can start by asking a few pertinent questions, taking care that this is done in a non-threatening manner. Should you establish that serious deficiencies in knowledge are present you must be flexible enough to try and correct them rather than ploughing on regardless into your prepared lecture.

Varying the format

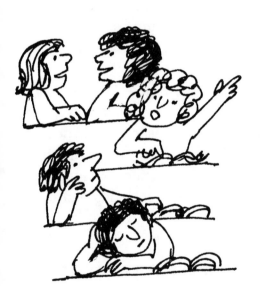

You must now give attention to the body of the lecture. Two main factors must be considered. Firstly, a purely verbal presentation will not be very effective and will contribute to a fall off in the level of arousal. You should therefore be planning ways of incorporating appropriate audiovisual aids. Secondly, the format of the lecture must be varied. Research studies have shown us that levels of arousal and learning will fall progressively. No more than twenty minutes should go by before the students are given a break or before the teaching technique is significantly altered. Ways of doing this include questioning or testing the students, generating discussion among students and showing a film or videotape segment. These are discussed in more detail in later sections.

Finishing the lecture

The conclusion of the lecture is as important as the introduction. Your closing comments should be well prepared. The last things that you say are the ones the students are most likely to remember. This will be the opportunity to reiterate the key points you hope to have made. You may also wish to direct students to additional reading at this time, but be reasonable in your expectations and give them a clear indication of what is essential as opposed to what you think is desirable. A couple of minutes to allow them to consolidate and read their notes is a worthwhile ploy.

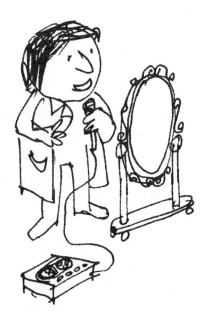

Rehearsal

Some of the best lecturers find it very helpful to rehearse so a dry run may be more important for the less experienced. However, the purpose of the rehearsal should not be to become word perfect. You must retain the flexibility to allow yourself to digress should the necessity occur. A rehearsal will often reveal that you are attempting to cram too much into the time and that some of your visual aids are poorly prepared or difficult to see from the rear of the theatre. The value of a rehearsal will be much enhanced if you invite along a colleague to act as the audience and to provide critical comments.

In some institutions you will have access to courses on teaching methods. Overcome your natural reluctance and enrol. It is likely that one component of the course will give you the opportunity of viewing your lecturing technique on videotape. The unit running the course may also provide an individual to come and observe your lecture, giving you the expert feedback you may not always get from a colleague.

Rehearsal may also give you the confidence to leave behind the full text of the lecture. (If you have the full text with you, you will be tempted to read it and thus ensure a rapid decline in levels of arousal.) Most good lecturers only bring with them a list of key points, often written on small pocket sized cards numbered in serial order. Others rely on slides and overhead transparencies to guide them.

WHAT ADDITIONAL TECHNIQUES ARE AVAILABLE?

We have already considered how variety in the presentation is essential in maintaining arousal. Even variety for variety's sake may be valuable but it is preferable to modify the format to match the varying purposes of the lecture. Ways of doing this may be categorized into variations in the manner and style of presentation, active participation of the students and use of audiovisual aids.

Variations in manner and style

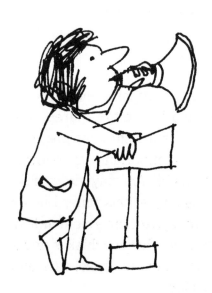

It is important that you feel comfortable with the way you present your lecture. However, you should not necessarily limit your manner and style to that of your basic personality. To maintain arousal and minimize the fall off in attention seen in Figure 1.1 you must vary your presentation. Changes in the volume and rate of speech, the use of silence, the maintenance of eye contact with the class and movement away from the lectern to create a less formal relationship should all be considered.

Active participation

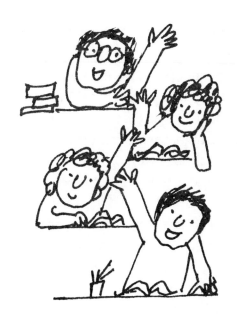

The most powerful way of enhancing learning is to devise situations which require the students to interact with yourself and with each other. **Questions** are the simplest form of interaction. Many lectures ask for questions at the end of their presentation but most are disappointed in the student response. Others direct questions at students during the lecture and this may be effective in producing a high level of arousal. However, unless the lecturer is very careful the dominant emotion may be one of fear. It is therefore preferable to engineer a situation in which all students answer the questions. You may wish to prepare the questions in the form of multiple-choice items which can be projected as slides or overhead transparencies. The class can be asked to indicate by show of hands which options they think are correct. Various more sophisticated ways to obtain such feedback from all students have been developed ranging from wiring all seats in the theatre with response buttons to issuing coloured response cards which are held up so only the lecturer can see the answers.

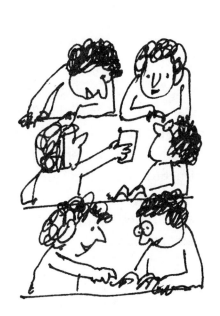

Small group activity should always be considered as it is a powerful teaching technique. Surprisingly, it is uncommonly attempted in the lecture situation even though it is simple to arrange for any number of students in any sized theatre. Once you try it out you may find it so exciting to hear the steady hum of students actually discussing your subject that you will never again feel comfortable giving a didactic lecture. The general approach is to break down the class into small groups, using a judicious rearrangement of seating if necessary. Small groups of 2–4 people may be formed among neighbours without any movement while larger groups may be quickly formed by 2–4 students in one row turning to form a group with students in the row behind. If a substantial amount of discussion time is planned the groups might best be formed at the beginning of the lecture and asked to spread themselves out to use up the whole lecture theatre space.

The selection of the most appropriate grouping will largely depend on what you wish to achieve. Small groups may be asked to discuss a limited topic for a few minutes (sometimes called buzz groups) or to consider broader topics for a longer period of time. You may then wish to allow all or some of the groups to report back to you. This is a very useful exercise when problems are given to the students to solve and where a variety of different responses can be expected.

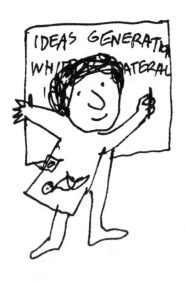

Brainstorming is a technique which can be modified for use in the lecture situation. It can be of value at the beginning of a lecture to stimulate interest in the topic to be discussed. The students are presented with an issue or problem and asked to contribute as many ideas or solutions as they can. All contributions are accepted without comment or judgement as to their merits and written on the blackboard or on an overhead transparency. This approach encourages 'lateral' or 'divergent' thinking. One of us has successfully used this technique with a class of 120 at the beginning of a lecture on the medical record. The session was commenced with a request for the class to put forward their suggestions as to the functions fulfilled by the record. These suggestions were then categorized and used as a basis for further discussion by the lecturer in an environment where the students had been the initiators of the discussion points.

One-to-one discussion is a particularly valuable technique in the situation where you might wish all the class to consider a very emotive or challenging concept. This method is described in detail in the chapter on small group teaching.

Use of audiovisual aids

The technical aspects of preparing and using audiovisual aids are discussed in detail in a separate chapter. This section will only cover those aspects pertinent to their use in the lecture situation. They may be used for a variety of purposes including illustrating the structure of the lecture, providing examples, stimulating interest and providing variety. The aids most likely to be used are overhead transparencies, slides, films or videotapes and demonstrations.

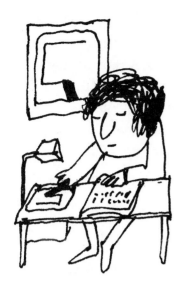

The overhead projector has largely replaced the blackboard in medical teaching. It has the advantages of allowing the lecturer to prepare material beforehand and to retain the information for future use. It also avoids the need to turn one's back to the audience. An overhead transparency is particularly useful for giving outlines and listing key points. A blank sheet of paper can be used to reveal the points in sequence. A pen or pencil placed on the transparency itself should be used to direct the students' attention to the appropriate point rather than using the pointer on the screen. Information may be added to the transparency as the lecture proceeds.

We have found that the value of the overhead is reduced by three common practices. Firstly, too much information is included on each transparency. Secondly, the lecturer works through the material too quickly or talks about something different while students are trying to read and take notes from the screen. Thirdly, the transparency is carelessly positioned or out of focus.

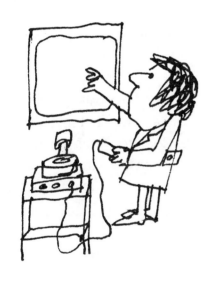

The 35mm slide is widely used and most lecturers build up an extensive collection. These are too often misused. In general, slides containing verbal material should be kept simple and must be clearly visible at the back of the theatre. Care must be taken when reproducing material from books and journals which often contain far too much material. Do not be guilty of introducing your slide with words such as 'this is a complex slide but I just want you to concentrate on this line of figures'. Coloured slides of patients, pathological specimens, X-rays and so on are ideal for illustrating didactic points and for adding variety and interest.

When using slides avoid turning off the lights for more than brief periods. The level of arousal will rapidly fall however interesting your slides happen to be.

Films and videotapes are best used in short segments. Their use requires more careful planning as it will be necessary to have a projectionist if a film is to be shown and probably a technician to set up video equipment. However, the effort is well worthwhile for both the impact of the content and the variety it introduces in the lecture. We use such material to show illustrative case histories, to demonstrate clinical situations infrequently seen on the wards (e.g. epileptic fits) and to show practical techniques. Film or videotapes may also be used in attempts to influence attitudes or to explore emotionally charged areas in the lecture setting. A short segment can be shown illustrating some challenging situation (trigger film) and the class asked to react to this situation. Films for this purpose are commercially available.

Handouts

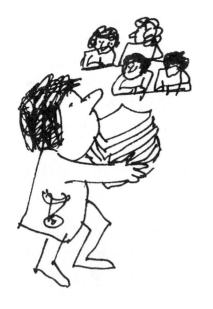

Little research has been done on the use of handouts but what has suggests that students get higher test scores from lectures accompanied by handouts, that students appreciate them and that the design of the handout influences note taking practices. One study showed that students preferred to write in the space between headings and the more space left, the more notes were taken.

Handouts may be valuable as a guide to the structure of the lecture and in this case may be very similar in content to the basic lecture plan. Such a handout should be given out at the beginning of a lecture.

You may wish to use the handout to provide detailed information on an area not well covered in standard student texts or not covered in detail during the lecture. Such handouts should be given out at the end of the lecture. Handouts may also be used to guide further study and to provide references for additional reading.

Student note taking

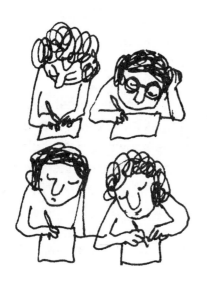

The research in this area generally supports the view that note taking should be encouraged. It is a process which requires the student to attend to the lecture. The process of encoding the information into the notes is one which aids its transfer into long term memory, particularly if students can be persuaded to read their notes shortly after the lecture is completed. The lecturer can assist this process by providing structures of material that is complex. Diagrams and other schematic representations may be more valuable than simple prose.

WHEN THINGS GO WRONG

Throughout this book we present the view that things are less likely to go wrong if you have carefully prepared yourself for the task. However, unexpected problems can and do arise so strategies to deal with these need to be part of your teaching skills.

In our experience problems are likely to fall into one of the following categories.

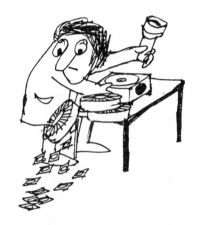

Problems with audio-visual materials and equipment

An equipment failure can be a potential disaster if you have prepared a series of slides or transparencies for projection. Preventive measures include having back-up equipment on hand, learning to change blown bulbs or removed jammed slides. If these measures are of no avail, you will have to continue on without the materials and may do so successfully provided you have taken care to have a clear record in your notes of the content of your slides or transparencies. Photocopied enlargements of slides of data are a useful back-up here. You may then be able to present some of the information verbally, on a blackboard or whiteboard or on an overhead transparency if the original problem was with the slide projector. You will not, of course, be able to use this approach with clinical illustrations and you may have to substitute careful description and perhaps blackboard sketches to cover essential material. Whatever you do, do not pass around your materials, which may be damaged and, of course, by the time most of the audience receives them, they are no longer directly relevant to what you are saying.

Problems with your presentation

Losing your place and running out of time can be disconcerting. Do not start apologizing or communicate your sense of 'panic' if these should happen. Instead, pause, calmly evaluate your situation, decide on a course of action and continue.

Problems with students

Tyro lecturers often fear confrontation with students in a lecture class. We cannot go into all aspects of classroom management and discipline here, but we can identify a number of principles and refer you to more detailed discussions elsewhere. (McKeachie's **Teaching Tips** is a useful reference.)

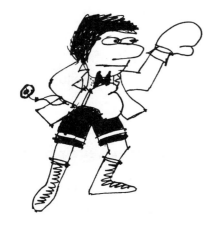

Disruptive behaviour and talking in class are common problems and must not be ignored, both for the sake of your own concentration and for the majority of students who are there to hear what you have to say. Minor disturbances can usually be overcome by simply stopping talking and waiting patiently for quiet. If this happens more than once the other students will usually make their displeasure made known to the offenders. If the disruption is more serious, you will have to speak directly to the students concerned and make them know you are aware of the offence. But do try initially to treat it with humour or you may alienate the rest of the class. If the problem persists, indicate you will be unable to tolerate the situation again and you will have to ask them to leave. Make sure you do just this if the problem re-emerges. Do so firmly and calmly. If the situation leads to confrontation, it is probably best if you leave yourself. It is remarkable what effect this has on disciplining a group of students! Make every attempt to meet the offenders afterwards to deal with the problem.

We have been appalled at accounts of lecturers who endure the most unreasonable physical and verbal abuse in lectures and do nothing about it – other than suffer inwardly. There is no need for this and the majority of students will respect firm and fair disciplinary measures.

EVALUATING THE LECTURE

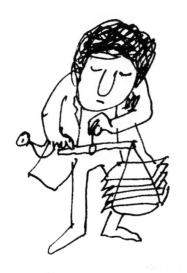

Improving the quality of your lecturing will depend on a combination of experience and your willingness to critically evaluate your performance. Evaluation may be seen as **informal** or **formal**. The informal way may involve asking one or two students whom you know for their comments. It may also be undertaken by asking yourself a series of questions immediately after the lecture.

- How much time was taken to prepare for the lecture?
- Were the notes helpful?
- Were the visual aids clear and easy to read?

- What steps could be taken to improve preparation and presentation?
- Did the questions stimulate discussion?
- Were the purposes of the presentation achieved?
- How did the students react?

The distribution of questionnaires to the class is a more formal way of evaluating a lecture. Many such forms have been designed and can usually be obtained from the teaching unit within your institution. An example of such a form designed by one of us is given overleaf. The questions asked have been derived from research on effective teaching. However, like all such forms its main limitation is that it cannot present answers to all the questions **you** may think are relevant. Accordingly, you should consider adding to or adapting such forms to your own special needs.

The best way of obtaining evaluation is to seek the services of a teaching unit. They will sit in on your lecture and prepare a detailed analysis. They might also suggest they record the presentation on video or audiotape and go back over it with you later.

GUIDED READING

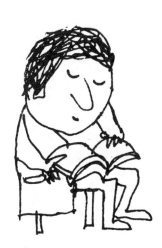

Almost all books which are concerned with the practicalities of teaching in education will devote some space to the lecture and you will undoubtedly find many of these helpful. Perhaps the most popular book on lecturing is Donald Bligh's *What's the Use of Lectures,* Penguin, 1972. Most libraries will have this publication which is, unfortunately, out of print. (A later edition is available from the author at Briar House, Clyst Honiton, Exeter EX5 2LZ, Devon, UK.) Bligh's book gives an overview of the research, useful information on preparing and delivering lectures and an interesting section on alternatives to the lecture.

A very practical book that can be recommended is George Brown's *Lecturing and Explaining,* Methuen, 1978. This book is full of exercises and suggested activities that you can carry out for yourself or with a colleague. Some chapter headings will suggest the flavour of this book: 'Learning to lecture', 'Preparing and designing explanations' and 'Helping students learn from lectures'.

STUDENT EVALUATION OF TEACHING

This questionnaire seeks information about your experience of *this* teacher and *this* course.

Please answer each question accurately. If you feel your cannot answer a particular question leave it out and go to the next question. Your responses are anonymous.

Circle the number which most closely corresponds to your view about each statement.

Thank you for your assistance with this evaluation.

COURSE .... LECTURER ....

PART A

1   How do you feel about the content of this course?

Very Positive	Positive	Neutral	Negative	Very Negative	
1	2	3	4	6	(1

2   *All things considered*, how would you rate this staff member's effectiveness as a university teacher?

Very Poor	Poor	Satisfactory	Good	Very Good
1	2	3	4	5

3   How would you describe the workload in this course?

Very Light	Light	Reasonable	Heavy	Very Heavy
1	2	3	4	5

4   The pace at which this course is being presented is . . .

Too Fast	Fast	About Right	Slow	Too Slow
1	2	3	4	5

5   How would you describe the degree of difficulty of this course?

Very Easy	Easy	Reasonable	Difficult	Very Difficult	
1	2	3	4	5	(5

PART B

Please indicate the extent to which you *agree or disagree* with the following statements by circling the appropriate number.

		Strongly Agree	Agree	Uncertain	Disagree	Strongly Disagree	
Course Characteristics							
6	I understand the subject matter	1	2	3	4	5	(6
7	This course is being *poorly* co-ordinated	1	2	3	4	5	
8	The course is challenging	1	2	3	4	5	
9	Assessment methods are fair	1	2	3	4	5	
10	Course materials are well prepared	1	2	3	4	5	
11	Proposed aims of course are being implemented	1	2	3	4	5	
12	I am learning something valuable	1	2	3	4	5	
13	Recommended readings contribute to understanding in the course	1	2	3	4	5	(13
Teacher Characteristics							
14	Communicates effectively	1	2	3	4	5	(14
15	Teaching style makes note-taking difficult	1	2	3	4	5	
16	Enthusiastic about teaching this course	1	2	3	4	5	
17	Stimulates my interest in this subject	1	2	3	4	5	
18	Interested in students	1	2	3	4	5	
19	Accessible to students outside classes	1	2	3	4	5	
20	Encourages students to express ideas	1	2	3	4	5	
21	Well organised	1	2	3	4	5	
22	Confident	1	2	3	4	5	
23	Clear explanations given	1	2	3	4	5	(23

PART C

24 What improvements to the course, or to the teaching, could you suggest?
Please PRINT your comments, to preserve anonymity, on the back of this sheet.

Thank you for answering this questionnaire. Please return it as directed.

From: *A Handbook for Medical Teachers*, Newble and Cannon, MTP Press, 1987

Books and journals referred to in this chapter:

Use Your Head by T. Buzan, BBC Publications, London, 1974.

Evaluating the Effectiveness of Lectures by B. Cooper and J. M. Foy, Universities Quarterly, 21, 1967.

Teaching Tips: A Guidebook for the Beginning College Teacher (7th edition) by W.J. McKeachie, Heath, Lexington, Massachusetts, 1978.

2: MAKING A PRESENTATION AT A SCIENTIFIC MEETING

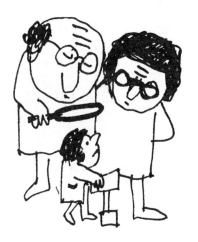

INTRODUCTION

This chapter may appear to be out of place in a book about education and teaching. However, most clinical teachers, at some time, will wish to make a presentation at a scientific meeting. There are many obvious similarities between giving a lecture and presenting a paper. There are also significant differences which may not be quite so obvious which made us feel that this chapter might be appreciated.

Poster sessions are growing in popularity at many national and international meetings as an alternative to the formal presentation of papers. We have, therefore, included a short segment on the preparation of a conference poster.

PRESENTING A PAPER

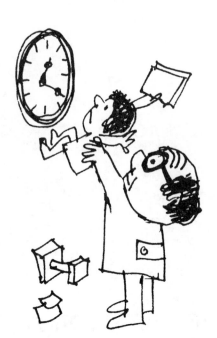

Though much of the advice given in the chapter on lecturing is just as relevant in this section, the aims of a scientific meeting or conference are different enough to warrant separate consideration. Much of this difference relates to the restriction on time. It is likely that a strict time limit of 10–15 minutes will be imposed. If you are in the position to give a paper it is certain you will have a lot to say, far more in fact than can possibly be delivered in such a short time. You will also be caught in the difficult situation of having many of the audience unfamiliar with the details of your area of interest, some of the audience knowing considerably more than you do about the area, and all of the audience likely to be critical of the content and the presentation. These and other factors make the giving of a scientific paper a pressure situation, particularly for the young and inexperienced lecturer hoping to make a good impression on his peers and superiors. However, it is also a situation that is amenable to resolution by careful planning and attention to technique.

PREPARING THE PAPER

Much of the advice that follows has been admirably dealt with previously by Calnan and Barabas in their excellent little book entitled *Speaking at Medical Meetings*. They describe three stages that you must go through during the preparation of a short scientific communication.

★ The collection and selection of the data.

★ The arrangement (getting the structure right and deciding on the most suitable visual aids).

★ Polishing, writing it out and rehearsal.

These same basic headings have been retained in this chapter.

The collection and selection of the data

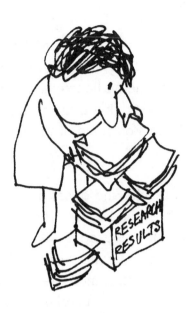

There is a great tendency for speakers to cram in more than is possible into their papers with the inevitable consequence of either speaking too fast or going over time. The audience knows that it is not possible to cross all the t's and dot all the i's and is primarily interested in hearing a short cohesive account of your research. To achieve this you are not going to be able to present all your hard won data. You are going to have to be very selective and in most instances you will have to restrict yourself to one aspect of your work.

Your first step should be to write down in one sentence the main purpose of your paper. In other words, what is the main message you wish to get across. Having done this you should identify the three or four pieces of evidence you will use to give support to your views. You should keep in mind that you will only have two to three minutes to describe each piece of work so that when you are assembling your data you must be aware of the need to simplify the results into a more easily digested form (e.g. complex tables reconstructed into histograms).

The arrangement

The first task is to get the basic plan worked out. The presentation will fall into several components.

● Introduction
● Statement of the purpose of your research
● Description of methods and results
● Conclusions

The introduction: this is a vital component of the talk. It must set the context of your work for the audience, many of whom may not be experts in your field. They may also be suffering the after effects of the previous paper or of a dash from another concurrent session venue. You have no more than two minutes to excite the interest of the audience before they relapse into the mental torpor so prevalent at medical meetings. You must therefore give a considerable amount of thought to the introduction. It must be simple, precise and free from jargon. It must start from a broad base so that the audience can identify the point at which your research fits into the scheme of things and make them appreciate the vital importance of your own contribution.

The statement of purpose: this should take no more than a minute but it is also a vital component of the talk. In these few sentences you will have to convince the audience that what you set out to do was worthwhile. It should flow from the introduction so that it sounds like a logical outcome of previous research.

The description of methods and results: the description of methods will usually have to be abbreviated or even reduced to a mention ('The so-and-so technique was used to . . .'). If the development of a new method is an important part of your work then it must obviously be described in more detail but you must decide whether the main message is to relate to the method or the results subsequently obtained.

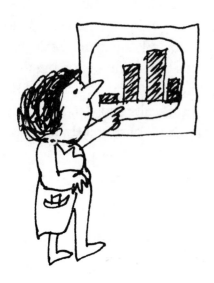

The results are usually the most important part of the paper. You will inevitably have spent a lot of time getting them together. It is possible that you have already prepared a variety of tables, graphs and charts for the purpose of publication. Do not fall into the trap of thinking that these are suitable for presentation to a live audience. How often have you, for example, sat in a meeting where someone has projected slides of an incomprehensible and illegible table taken straight from a journal!

The conclusions: this must flow naturally from the results of your work. You will be aiming to make one or two clear statements which you are able to make from your work. It is advisable to be reasonably modest in your claims.

The visual aids: the second task is to prepare the visual aids. In most instances these will be slides or overhead transparencies. Considerable thought must be given to these as their impact and quality may make or break the presentation. They must complement your oral presentation, not duplicate it. The technical aspects of the preparation of slides and overhead transparencies are covered in greater detail in the chapter dealing with teaching aids but a few specific points are worth mentioning at this time.

Having roughed out the plan of the talk it should be reasonably obvious where a slide is required. You may need one or two during the introduction, such as a clinical picture of a patient or an illustration of a previous piece of research. You may not have time to say much about the method but a slide illustrating the technique may be pertinent. If so, simple line diagrams are usually more valuable than photographs.

The slides of the results provide you with the greatest challenge. It is during this part of your paper that the visual material will often be of more importance than the verbal ('A picture says a thousand words'). Avoid complex tables and where possible convert tables to charts or simple graphs. Rarely is it appropriate to show masses of individual data; just show the mean or rounded off figures. If you feel you really must refer to complex data it is better to have this prepared in printed form and distributed to the audience.

Having prepared the slides, check that they are accurate and legible (as a rough rule a slide where the information can be read with the naked eye will be satisfactory when projected). Then take them to a large lecture theatre and project them. Check that they are indeed legible from the furthermost corners of the theatre. It is also helpful to take a colleague with you to check that the message is clear and that there are no spelling mistakes.

Polishing, writing it out and rehearsal

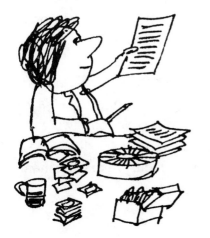

At this stage you should have a good idea of what you intend to say and the visual aids that you require. It is now advisable to write the text of the talk in full. Do not write in the style you use for journal publications. Pretend you are talking to an individual and write in a conversational mode, avoiding jargon wherever possible. As you go along identify the correct position for the slides. You may find places where you have not prepared an appropriate slide. This should be rectified even if the slide is only to consist of a couple of key words.

Remember, during the talk the slides must complement your talk and not distract from it. There must always be an accurate match between the content of your slide and what you are saying. If you do not have a slide to illustrate what you are saying, insert a blank slide rather than leaving on an irrelevant slide. This will also avoid the distracting practice of saying 'slide-off' and 'slide-on'. If you intend to use the same slide more than once get multiple copies made to avoid the confusion that will ensue if you ask the projectionist to go back to a previous slide.

Once you have the rough draft, edit it. Then read it aloud at about the pace you think you will go during the presentation. Further editing and alterations will be required as almost certainly you will have gone over time. Some find it a useful ploy at this stage to record the talk on a tape recorder and listen to the result very critically.

The next stage is to present the paper (including the slides) to an honest and critical colleague. The feedback is often extremely valuable. At this stage you will have finalized the text and slides.

You must now make the decision whether you will read the paper or not. Most authorities consider that you should be well enough rehearsed to speak only with the aid of cue cards or the cues provided by your slides. If you have a highly visual presentation most of the audience will be looking at the screen so the fact that you are reading is less critical. Providing the text is written in a conversational style, and you are able to look up from your text at frequent intervals, then reading is not a major sin. The chief risk of speaking without a text in a very short presentation is going over time which at best will irritate the chairman and the audience, and at worst will result in your being cut off in mid sentence.

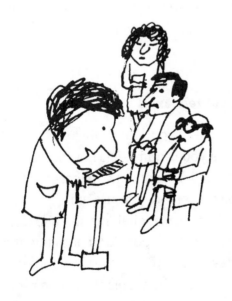

Whatever you decide, rehearsal is essential and a dress rehearsal in front of an audience (e.g. the Department) a week or two before the event is invaluable. Not only will you receive comments on the presentation but you will also be subject to questions, the answering of which, in a precise manner, is just as important as the talk itself.

PREPARING THE ABSTRACT AND YOUR CONTRIBUTION TO THE PROCEEDINGS OF THE CONFERENCE

The abstract

Most conferences will require you to prepare an abstract, sometimes several months before the meeting. It may initially be used to help select contributions and will ultimately be made available to participants. Contributors are often tardy in preparing their abstracts which is discourteous to the conference organizers and makes their task more difficult.

The abstract should be an advertisement for your paper. It should outline the background to the study (very similar to the introductory section of your paper) and summarize the supporting data and the main conclusions. Quite frequently abstracts promise what they do not deliver so avoid becoming guilty of false advertising.

The proceedings

Many national and most major international conferences will publish proceedings. Should you be presenting a paper at such a conference you will be required to provide your contribution to these proceedings during the conference or shortly afterwards. It is not appropriate to present the organizers with the script and slides that you have just used in your presentation. The contribution to the proceedings should be written in a style consistent with that used in a journal article. The content should be the same as in the presented paper but not necessarily identical. It is perfectly permissible to expand some areas, particularly with regard to the methods and results sections, where more detail could be included. This should, of course, all be done within the guidelines for format and length specified by the organizers.

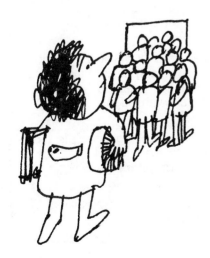

WHAT YOU SHOULD DO ON THE DAY

'There's many a slip twixt cup and lip.' This saying provides a reminder that, however good your preparation for the presentation of the paper has been, there is still plenty that can happen to ruin your carefully laid plans. Fortunately, many such problems can be prevented or anticipated. You should find it helpful to work your way through this checklist.

FIGURE 2·1
CHECKLIST TO USE ON
THE DAY OF THE
PRESENTATION

Before the presentation:

★ Check your slides to see that they are in the correct order, labelled in this order and spotted in the correct place (see Fig. 7.5).

★ If possible, load your slides into an empty magazine of the type to be used during your presentation. Project them somewhere to check that they are indeed in the correct order and the right way around. Then seal the magazine and label it with your name.

★ Seek out the projectionist and explain your plan for the slides and the arrangements for lighting.

★ Check your prompt cards or text.

★ Check the venue and audiovisual facilities. You may be expected to operate the lights, a slide changer and a light pointer. Have a practice during a break in the programme.

★ If you are expected to use a microphone check how it is attached or adjusted.

★ Try and sit in on a talk in the same venue early in the day to get a feel for the acoustics and how you should use the audiovisual facilities.

During the presentation:

● Walk confidently to the podium and arrange your cards or text. Adjust the microphone and set out the position of pointers, slide changers and so on to your satisfaction.

● Commence your talk with an appropriate opening ('Mr Chairman, ladies and gentlemen').

● Present the opening few sentences without reference to any notes, looking around the audience without fixing your eye on any particular individual, however friendly or prestigious that person may be.

● Call for the lights to be dimmed (or do it yourself) when your first slide is to appear. Never turn off the lights completely unless it is absolutely essential and in any case only for a minimum of time. On the other hand do not continually call for 'lights on' or 'lights off'. Your slides should have been designed to be clearly visible in subdued light.

● Speak at a rate which sounds slow to you – it will not be too slow for the audience. Try and use more emphasis than seems natural to your own ear – again, it will not sound too theatrical to the audience. Let your enthusiasm show through by using suitable hand and facial gestures.

● When you turn to the screen to point something out on the slide make sure you do not move away from the microphone. This is a particular problem with a fixed microphone, in which case move behind it so you continue to speak across it.

● When you come to the conclusion, say so ('In conclusion, Mr Chairman, I have shown ...'. 'Finally, ...').

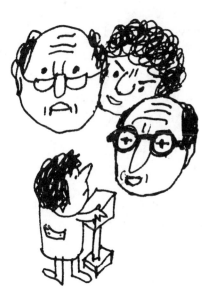

FIGURE 2·2
POINTS TO REMEMBER
WHEN HANDLING
QUESTIONS

Handling questions

Most conferences have a fixed period of time for questions. In some ways this is the most critical part of the presentation. Some people in the audience are going to test you out with penetrating questions and how you handle them will enhance or detract from the impact of your performance. This is one of the reasons why we suggested a full dress rehearsal in front of your Department in order to practice your answering of difficult questions and to avoid leaving weaknesses in your arguments for which some participants will be eagerly searching. The following are some points to remember:

★ Listen to the question very carefully.

★ If the question is complex or if you suspect that not all the audience heard it, restate it clearly and succinctly.

★ Answer the question politely and precisely. Sometimes a simple 'yes' or 'no' will be sufficient. Avoid the danger of using the question to give what amounts to a second paper.

★ Be alert to the questioner who is deliberately trying to trick you or to use the occasion to display his own knowledge of the subject.

★ If the question is particularly awkward or aggressive try to deflect it as best you can. Strategies include agreeing with as much of what was said as possible, acknowledging legitimate differences of opinion or interpretation, or suggesting you meet the questioner afterwards to clarify your position. At all costs avoid a heated head-on clash in front of your audience. However, do not be afraid to politely disagree with any questioners, however eminent, when you are sure of your ground. Remember, they may only be testing you out.

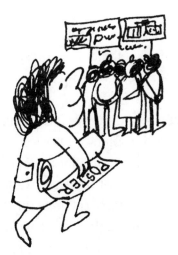

PREPARING A CONFERENCE POSTER

The conference poster is an increasingly popular alternative to presenting papers at conferences. You will find that the poster has several advantages over the traditional paper such as:

⇒ allowing readers to consider material at their own rate;

⇒ being available for viewing over an extended period of time;

⇒ enabling participants to engage in more detailed discussion with the presenter than is the case with the usually rushed paper discussion session.

If the conference organizers have arranged a poster session we suggest that you consider taking advantage of it. It may provide you with an opportunity to present additional material to the conference that would otherwise be difficult because of limitations on the number of speakers.

What is a conference poster?

A conference poster is a means of presenting information from a static display. A poster should include at least the following parts:

★ A title
★ An abstract
★ Text and diagrams
★ Name of author(s), their address(es) and where they may be contacted during the conference.

Additional material that you might consider for the poster, or in support of the poster, include:

● Illustrations
● Exhibits and objects
● Audiovisual displays, such as a synchronized tape-slide presentation or videotape
● A take-away handout, which might be a printed reduction of your poster
● A blank pad, so that when you are not in attendance interested readers can leave comments or contact addresses for follow-up.

Preparing the poster

If you decide that a poster is an appropriate way of presenting your information, there are a number of things you must take into consideration during its preparation.

Firstly, ascertain from the conference organizers the facilities that will be available. Then proceed to plan the poster. The poster should communicate your message as simply as possible, so do not allow it to become clogged with too much detail. Layout ideas can be gleaned by looking through newspapers and magazines or, better still, from graphic design books and journals. If possible, discuss these ideas with a medical or graphic artist. The layout should be clear, logical and suitable for the material being presented. Try a number of different rough layouts first and seek the opinion of a colleague to determine the best.

FIGURE 2.3

POSSIBLE LAYOUT FOR A CONFERENCE POSTER

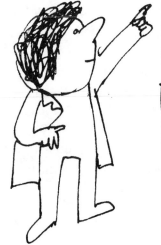

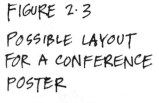

Text lettering should be large enough to be read at the viewing distance, which is likely to be about one metre. In this case, we suggest that the smallest letters be at least 5mm high and preferably larger. Titles can be prepared using Letraset or on a lettering machine that produces large and bold characters. For detailed text, a clear typewritten sheet prepared on a good quality electric typewriter can be photographically enlarged. Make sure diagrams are bold enough to be seen easily and consider using colour to highlight significant points.

Break up the density of text into several discrete parts. For example, consider dividing the text into an abstract, an introduction, a statement of method, results and conclusion – each with its own clear heading. A short list of references or of publications arising out of your work might also be appropriate. Remember, that in preparing your poster you are really trying to achieve many of the same things you would wish to achieve with a talk or lecture: attract attention, maintain interest and generally communicate effectively.

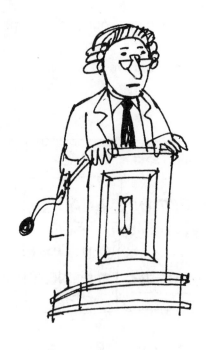

CHAIRING A CONFERENCE SESSION

Much of the success of a conference will depend on the quality of the chairmanship of individual sessions. Should this task fall to you, there are many responsibilities to fulfil. There are three categories of tasks – responsibilities to the organizers, to the speaker and to the audience.

Responsibilities to the organizers

The organizers of the conference will have approached you several months before the event. If you are lucky, they will also have given you detailed guidelines to follow but if not you must, at a minimum, find out:

★ The time and length of the session.
★ The number and names of the speakers.
★ A copy of the instructions given to speakers with particular reference to the time allocated for the presentation and the time allocated for discussion.
★ Whether they are concurrent sessions.

The ideal chairman will contact the speakers in advance of the conference to ensure they have indeed received instructions and understand their implications, particularly with regard to time. You may find that some are inexperienced and nervous about the prospect of their presentation and your advice will be appreciated. Referring the speaker to the earlier parts of this chapter might be valuable.

If early contact has not been made, it is essential to meet with speakers prior to the session. You must clarify the format of the session and reinforce your intention to stick rigidly to the allocated time. You should explain the method to be used to indicate when there is one minute to go, when time is up and what steps you will take should the speaker continue for longer than 10–15 seconds over time. This may sound draconian but, believe us, it is vital. A timing device on the lectern is an invaluable aid to compliance.

Prior to the session, you must also familiarize yourself with the layout of the venue, the audio-visual facilities and the lighting. In the absence of a technician, you may be called on to operate the equipment and lighting or to instruct the speakers in how to do so.

At the start of the session, announce that you intend to keep to time – and do so.

Finally, you must be certain that the session and individual presentations commence and finish at the programmed time. This is particularly important when there are concurrent sessions.

Responsibilities to the speakers

Speakers invariably fall into one of three types:

The well-organized speakers: they will tell **you** exactly what they are going to do and what they require. If you ask them how long they are going to speak, they will tell you in minutes and seconds! You will need to have little concern for these speakers, but they will expect you to be as well-prepared and organized as themselves.

The apprehensive speakers: they will generally be the younger and less experienced. They will often have a well-prepared paper to present but are in danger of not doing themselves justice. You can assist such speakers greatly by familiarizing them with the facilities before the session and encouraging them to practice operating the audio-visual equipment. If this seems beyond them, you may be able to take on this task yourself. Calm reassurance that all will be well is the message to convey.

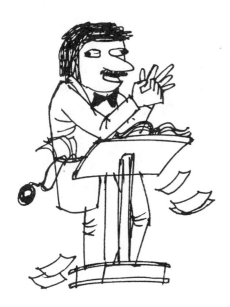

The confident underprepared speakers: these are remarkably prevalent and the most dangerous for the chairman. They will not seek advice and will deny having received detailed instructions about their presentation. When you ask them how long they expect to speak, you will receive an off-hand response. This will tell you they have not rehearsed their presentation and will almost certainly go over time. There is little you can do to help such people because they are certain they have everything under control. However, they can be your downfall unless you prepare to intervene. Prior to the session you must convince them you are serious about cutting them off if they speak over time. Unfortunately this strategy will often fail and you must be prepared to act immediately the first time a speaker goes over the allotted time. After a maximum of 15 seconds grace rise from your chair. If the hint is not immediately taken, you have no option but to politely but firmly stop the speaker. Examples can be cited of such speakers being physically led off the stage still talking, but such extremes should not arise. Fortunately, you will only have to intervene in such a way once in a session and, should it happen, your future as an invited chairman is assured.

In the discussion period you must see fair play. Ensure that questions are relevant and brief. Do not allow a questioner to make long statements or commence a mini-presentation of their own work. Suggest any significant differences of opinion be explored informally at the subsequent coffee break.

Responsibilities to the audience

The audience has a right to expect several things of the chairman. They must be able to hear the speaker and see any slides. They must be reassured that you will keep the speakers to time to protect their opportunity to ask questions. Speakers going over time is the commonest complaint of participants and the chairman is usually held to blame. During the question period you should ensure that the time is not monopolized by the intellectual heavies in the front rows. On the other hand you must also be prepared to ask the first question if none are immediately forthcoming from the audience.

Finishing off

At the close of the session, thank the speakers and the audience. Also remind them of the starting time of the next session. You may also have been asked to transmit information from the organizers. Particularly important would be to obtain completed evaluation forms for the session if these had been provided.

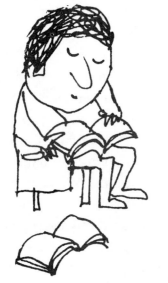

GUIDED READING

The book we recommend for further reading is Calnan and Barabas' *Speaking at Medical Meetings*, Heinemann, London, 1972. This pocket sized do-it-yourself guide is not only valuable but entertaining. It also contains many useful illustrations and good advice about the preparation of visual aids.

Those interested in the organization and evaluation of medical meetings are referred to a series entitled *Improving Medical Meetings*, writted by D.E. Richmond and his colleagues, published in the British Medical Journal, **287**, 1983, pp. 1201–2; 1286–7; 1363–4; 1450–1.

With regard to the preparation of posters, a useful reference is *Static Displays – Posters, Wallcharts, Exhibits in Medical Education*, Council for Educational Technology, London, 1973.

An excellent general text on public speaking is C. Turk, *Effective Speaking*, Spon, London, 1985. This is a comprehensive reference work that has been written by a university lecturer. You should consider obtaining a copy for your personal library. It is easy to use and very helpful.

3: TEACHING IN SMALL GROUPS

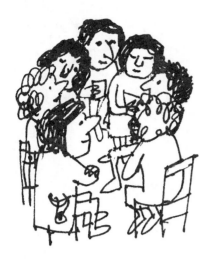

INTRODUCTION

This chapter assumes you have been asked to teach a small group. It also assumes that the group you are to take will meet on more than one occasion and therefore will present you with the opportunity to establish and develop a productive group atmosphere. Small group teaching can be a most rewarding experience. However, to achieve success you will need to plan carefully and to develop skills in group management. You should not fall into the common error of believing that discussion in groups will just happen. Even if it does, it is often directionless, unproductive, unsatisfying and perhaps threatening. To avoid these problems you will need some understanding of how groups work and how to apply a range of small group techniques to achieve the goals you set out to achieve.

THE IMPORTANCE OF SMALL GROUP TEACHING

Teaching in small groups enjoys an important place among the teaching methods commonly found in medical education for two rather different reasons. The first of these can be described as **social** and the other as **educational**. For many students in the university, and especially those in the early years of their studies, the small group or tutorial provides an important social contact with peers and teachers. The value of this contact should not be underestimated as a means for students to meet and deal with people and to resolve a range of matters indirectly associated with your teaching, such as difficulties with studying, course attendance and so on. Such matters will, of course, assist with the attainment of the more strictly educational objectives of your course.

Among the educational objectives that you can best achieve through the use of small group teaching methods are the development of higher-level intellectual skills such as reasoning and problem-solving, the development of attitudes and the acquisition of interpersonal skills such as listening, speaking, arguing, and group leadership. These skills are important to medical students who will eventually become involved professionally with patients, other health care professionals, community groups, learned societies and the like. The distinction between social and educational aspects of small group teaching is rather an arbitrary one but it is important to bear it in mind when you plan for small group teaching.

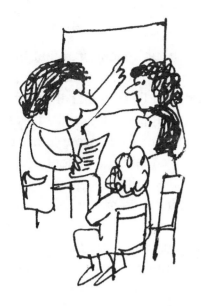

WHAT IS SMALL GROUP TEACHING?

Much of what passes for small group teaching in medical schools turns out to be little more than a lecture to a small number of students. Nor is size, within limits, a critical feature for effective small group teaching. We believe that small group teaching must have at least the following three characteristics:

- active participation
- face-to-face contact
- purposeful activity.

Active participation

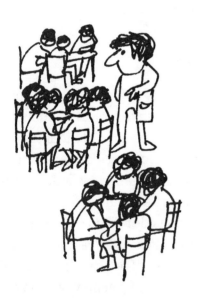

The first, and perhaps the most important, characteristic of small group teaching is that teaching and learning is brought about through discussion among **all** present. This generally implies a group size that is sufficiently small to enable each group member time to contribute. Research and practical experience has established that between five and eight students is ideal for most small group teaching. You will know, from experience, that many so-called small groups or tutorial groups are very much larger than this ideal. Although a group of over twenty students hardly qualifies as a small group it is worth remembering that, with a little ingenuity, you can use many of the small group teaching procedures described in this chapter with considerable success with larger numbers of students. Generally speaking, though, you will be looking for a technique which allows you to break the number down into subgroups for at least some of the time.

Face-to-face contact

The second characteristic of small group teaching is that it involves face-to-face contact among all those present. You will find it difficult to conduct satisfactory small group teaching in a lecture theatre or tutorial room with students sitting in rows. Similarly, long boardroom-type tables are quite unsuitable because those present cannot see all other group members, especially those seated alongside. Effective discussion requires communication which is not only verbal but also non-verbal involving, for example, gestures, facial expressions, eye contact and posture. This will only be achieved by sitting the group in a circle.

Purposeful activity

The third characteristic of small group teaching is that the session must have a purpose and must develop in an orderly way. It is certainly not an occasion for idle chit-chat although, regrettably, some teaching in groups appears to be little more than this. The purposes you set for your small group can be quite wide. They include discussing a topic or a patient problem and developing skills such as a criticizing, analysing, problem-solving and decision making. It is highly likely that you will wish the small group session to achieve more than one purpose. In medical schools, most groups are expected to deal with a substantial amount of content. However, you will also wish to use the small group approach to develop the higher intellectual skills of your students and even to influence their attitudes. In order to achieve these various purposes you will need considerable skills in managing the group and a clear plan so that the discussion will proceed in an orderly fashion towards its conclusion.

MANAGING A SMALL GROUP

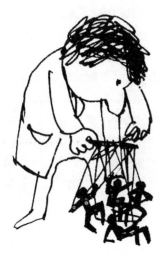

Small group teaching is considerably more difficult to manage than a lecture because you must take a closer account of the students' behaviour, personalities and difficulties. To achieve success with a small group you must also have a clear understanding of how a group operates and how it develops. You have particular responsibilities as the initial leader of the group but your role will vary considerably, both within a session and from session to session. For instance, if you adopt an autocratic or authoritarian style of leadership (not an uncommon one among clinical teachers) you may well have a lot of purposeful activity but there will be a limited amount of spontaneous participation. You should preferably adopt a role which is a more co-operative one where you demonstrate an expectation that the students will take responsibility for initiating discussion, providing information, asking questions, challenging statements, asking for clarification and so on. A successful group is one that can proceed purposefully without the need for constant intervention by the teacher. This is hard for most teachers to accept but is very rewarding if one recognizes that this independence is one of the key goals of small group teaching and is more important than satisfying one's own need to be deferred to as teacher and content expert.

In managing a group there are two main factors that have to be considered. These are those relating to the **task** of the group and those relating to the **maintenance** of the group. In addition there must be a concern for the needs of each student within the group.

The tasks of the group: These must be clearly defined. This is something that must be high on the agenda of the first meeting. The reason for the small group sessions and their purpose in the course must be explained. In addition, you must initiate a discussion about how you wish the group to operate, what degree of preparation you expect between group meetings, what role you intend to adopt, what roles you expect the students to assume and so on. Because such details may be quickly forgotten it is desirable to provide the student with a handout. The following list of headings may be helpful:

FIGURE 3.1
SUGGESTED HEADINGS FOR
A SMALL GROUP HANDOUT

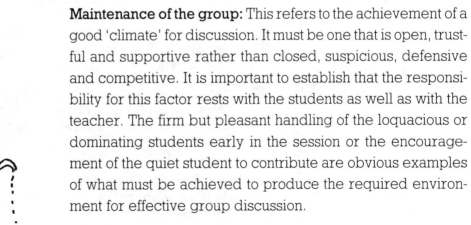

- Course title, description and aims
- Teacher's name and availability
- List of students' names
- How the group is to run (e.g. teacher's role, students' roles, method to be used)
- Work requirements (e.g. assignments, case presentations)
- Assessment arrangements
- Reading matter

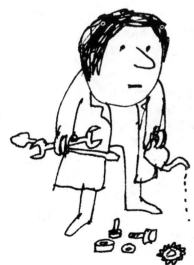

Maintenance of the group: This refers to the achievement of a good 'climate' for discussion. It must be one that is open, trustful and supportive rather than closed, suspicious, defensive and competitive. It is important to establish that the responsibility for this factor rests with the students as well as with the teacher. The firm but pleasant handling of the loquacious or dominating students early in the session or the encouragement of the quiet student to contribute are obvious examples of what must be achieved to produce the required environment for effective group discussion.

The successfully managed group will meet the following criteria:

41

FIGURE 3·2
CRITERIA FOR A GOOD GROUP
(AFTER HILL, 1982)

- Prevalence of a warm, accepting, non-threatening group climate.
- Learning approached as a co-operative rather than a competitive enterprise.
- Learning accepted as the major reason for the existence of the group.
- Active participation by all.
- Equal distribution of leadership functions.
- Group sessions and learning tasks are enjoyable.
- Content adequately and efficiently covered.
- Evaluation accepted as an integral part of the group's activities.
- Students attend regularly.
- Students come prepared.

STRUCTURE IN SMALL GROUP TEACHING

We mentioned earlier the need to have a clear plan so that the group discussion will proceed with purpose and in an orderly fashion. A structured approach to the task and the allocation of the time available is a useful tool for you to consider. An example of such a structured discussion session is illustrated in Figure 3.3.

FIGURE 3·3
STRUCTURED CASE
DISCUSSION SESSION

1	PRELIMINARIES/HOUSEKEEPING MATTERS	5 MINS
2	A STUDENT PRESENTS THE INITIAL HISTORY AND EXAMINATION FINDING OF ONE OF HIS WARD PATIENTS	5 MINS
3	GROUP ASKED TO GENERATE HYPOTHESES AND DIAGNOSES, DISCUSS IMMEDIATE MANAGEMENT AND INITIAL INVESTIGATIONS	15 MINS
4	INFORMATION PROVIDED ON WHAT THE STUDENT (AND CONSULTANT) THOUGHT WAS THE DIAGNOSIS, WHAT WAS DONE, AND WHICH INVESTIGATIONS WERE ORDERED. GROUP DISCUSSES ANY DISPARITIES	10 MINS
5	STUDENT PRESENTS FURTHER DATA ON INVESTIGATIONS AND PROGRESS. GROUP DISCUSSES ANY DISPARITIES	10 MINS
6	GROUP LEADER OFFERS CONCLUDING REMARKS AND OPPORTUNITY FOR CLARIFICATION OF UNRESOLVED ISSUES	5 MINS
	TOTAL	50 MINS

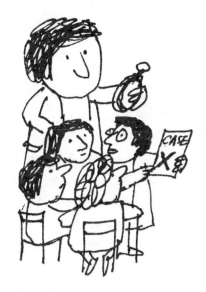

This is a structure of a discussion based on a case presentation. Note that the structure lays out **what** is to be discussed and how much **time** is budgeted. Such a scheme is not intended to encourage undue rigidity or inflexibility, but to clarify purposes and tasks. This may seem to be a trivial matter, but it is one which creates considerable uncertainty for students. Keeping to a time budget is very difficult. You need to be alert to how time is being spent and whether time from one part of the plan can be transferred to an unexpected and important issue that arises during discussion.

Another structure, not commonly used in medical education is illustrated in Figure 3.4.

FIGURE 3.4

A SNOWBALLING GROUP DISCUSSION (AFTER NORTHEDGE)

INDIVIDUAL WORK   10 MINS

STUDENTS READ BRIEF BACKGROUND DOCUMENT ON TOPIC, READ CASE HISTORY AND EXAMINE LABORATORY RESULTS.

WORK IN PAIRS   10 MINS

STUDENTS COMPARE UNDERSTANDINGS, CLEAR UP DIFFICULTIES, MAKE PRELIMINARY DIAGNOSIS AN DECIDE ON FURTHER TESTS

WORK IN SMALL GROUP   15 MINS

PAIRS REPORT TO THE SMALL GROUP. GROUP DISCUSSES DIAGNOSES AND FURTHER TESTS, SEEKING AGREEMENT OR CLARIFYING DIS-AGREEMENTS. GROUP PREPARES REPORT FOR WHOLE GROUP

REPORTING BACK TO WHOLE GROUP   20 MINS

EACH SMALL GROUP PRESENTS REPORT. TEACHER NOTES MAIN POINTS ON BOARD, BUTCHERS PAPER OR OVERHEAD TRANSPARENCY. AS GROUPS CON-TRIBUTE, TEACHER AND STUDENTS OFFER COM-MENTS. TEACHER OR STUDENTS ATTEMPT SUM-MARY OF POINTS RAISED AND SOME FORM OF CONCLUSION.

This structure includes the principle of 'snow-balling' groups. From an individual task, the student progresses through a series of small groups of steadily increasing size. There are special advantages in using this structure which are worth noting: it does not depend on prior student preparation for its success; the initial individual work brings all students to approximately the same level before discussion begins; and it ensures that everyone participates, at least in the preliminary stages.

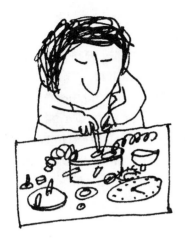

WHEN THINGS GO WRONG

You will undoubtedly have a variety of difficulties to deal with in your group sessions. For example, you might decide to ignore a sleeping student or an amorous couple in a lecture class, providing it was not disruptive, but it would be impossible to do so in a small group. How you resolve problems with the working of the group is critical. An authoritarian approach would almost certainly destroy any chance of establishing the co-operative climate we believe to be essential. It is generally more appropriate to raise the problem with the group and ask them for their help with a solution.

One of your main roles as a group leader is to be sensitive to the group and the individuals within it. Research has identified a number of difficulties that students commonly experience. These are connected with:

★ making a contribution to the discussion
★ understanding the conventions of group work and acceptable modes of behaviour
★ knowing enough to contribute to the discussion being assessed.

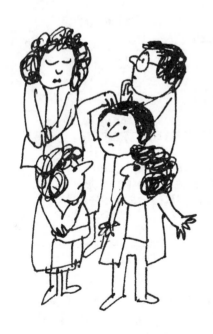

These difficulties frequently get in the way of productive discussion. They tend to be due to genuine confusion on the part of students combined with a fear of exposing their ignorance in front of the teacher and their peers. It is therefore essential for you to clarify the purpose of the group and the way in which students are to enter into the discussion. Their previous experience of small group sessions or ward teaching might lead them to see the occasion as only a threatening question and answer session. They must learn that ignorance is a relative term and that their degree of ignorance must be recognized and explored before effective learning can begin. A willingness by the teacher to admit his own ignorance and demonstrate an appropriate way of dealing with it will be very reassuring to many students.

Confusion in the students' minds about how they are being assessed can also cause difficulties. Generally speaking, assessing contributions to discussion is inhibiting and should be avoided if possible. If you do not have discretion in this matter then at least make it quite clear what criteria you are looking for in your assessment. Should you be able to determine your own assessment policy then the following are worth considering:

➡ require attendance at all (or a specified proportion of) group meetings as a prerequisite;

➡ set formal written work, e.g. a major essay, a series of short papers, a case analysis;

➡ set a group-based task, e.g. keeping an account of the work done by the group.

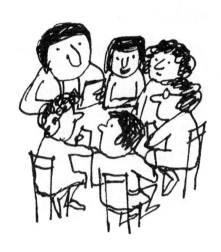

The teacher's perceptions of group difficulties may not necessarily match those of the students. A discussion with the group about how they think things are going or the administration of a short questionnaire are ways of seeking feedback.

Once the group is operating it is important to be continually on the look out for trouble. You must be sensitive to the emotional responses of the group and to the behaviour of individual students. Bion has categorized group responses into fight, flight, pairing and dependency. These categories serve to highlight some of the common features in groups which hinder their successful operation.

Fight: this appears in several forms. It may be easily recognized as overt hostility and aggression but equally damaging can be misplaced humour, quibbling over semantics, point scoring and attempting to establish intellectual superiority. Teachers are as frequently guilty of such activities as their students.

Flight: students become very adept at avoiding difficult situations. In our experience this is one of the biggest problems in small groups. It may take the form of withdrawal from active participation, by distracting behaviour, or by attempting to change the direction of the discussion without the resolution of a sticky problem.

Pairing: a pair within the group may carry on a more or less personal conversation for considerable periods of time. All too often the teacher is one of them. A good group will not allow this but in many groups the majority of the discussion may be carried on by only a small minority of students.

Dependency: this is also a common problem and is one which may be present in a whole group. The group avoids tackling problems by getting someone to do it for them. This may be the brightest student or most frequently the teacher who may even be flattered into it. Medical students seem to be particularly adept at this and their teachers particularly susceptible.

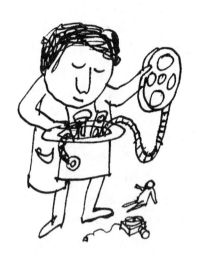

INTRODUCING STIMULUS MATERIALS

A very useful means of getting discussion going in groups is to use what is generally known as 'stimulus material'. We have seen how this was done in the snowballing group structure described previously. The range of stimulus material is really very large indeed. It is limited only by your imagination and the objectives of your course. Here are a few examples:

- a short multiple-choice test (ambiguous items work well in small groups)
- a case history
- a trigger film or video (e.g. short open-ended situation, such as a patient's reaction to a doctor)
- a patient
- observation of a role-play
- visual materials (e.g. X-rays, photographs, slides, specimens, real objects, charts, diagrams, statistical data)
- an audio recording (e.g. an interview, heart sounds, a segment of a radio broadcast)
- a student's written report on a project or a patient
- a patient management problem or modified essay question (see Chapter 6)
- a journal article or other written material

One of the most innovative approaches we have encountered was that developed by Moore at the University of Melbourne. He used extracts from literary works to help students understand the broader cultural, philosophical, ethical and personal issues of being a doctor. Examples of sources for these extracts include Solzhenitsyn's **Cancer Ward** and Virginia Woolf's **On Being Ill.**

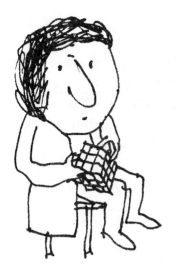

ALTERNATIVE SMALL GROUP DISCUSSION TECHNIQUES

As with any other aspect of teaching it is helpful to have a variety of techniques at one's fingertips in order to introduce variety or to suit a particular situation. Such techniques include:

★ One-to-one discussion
★ Buzz groups
★ Brainstorming
★ Role playing
★ Evaluation discussion

1. One-to-one discussion

This is a very effective technique which can be used with a group of almost any size. It is particularly useful as an 'ice breaker' when the group first meets, and is valuable for enhancing listening skills. It can also be used to discuss controversial or ethical issues when forceful individuals with strong opinions will be prevented from dominating the discussion. They will also be required to listen to other opinions and express them to the whole group.

FIGURE 3·5
CONDUCTING A ONE-TO-ONE
DISCUSSION

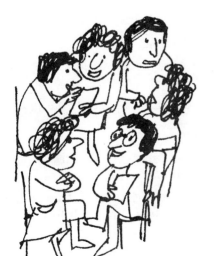

A Procedure
- group members (including the teacher) divide into pairs and each person is designated 'A' or 'B'
- person A talks to person B for an **uninterrupted** period of 3–5 minutes on the topic for discussion.
- person B listens and avoids prompting or questioning.
- roles are reversed with B talking to A.
- at the conclusion the group reassembles.
- each person, in turn, introduces themselves before introducing the person to whom they were speaking. They then briefly paraphrase what was said by that person.

B Use as icebreaker
- group members are asked to respond to a question such as 'tell me something about yourself'.

C General use
- group members respond to appropriate questioning, e.g. 'what is your opinion about...?'

It can be useful to insist on the no interruption rule (though not so much when used as an icebreaker). Prolonged periods of silence may ensue but person A will be using this time for uninterrupted thinking, a luxury not available in most situations. Often the first superficial response to a question will be changed after deeper consideration.

2. Buzz groups

These are particularly helpful to encourage maximum participation at one time. It is therefore especially useful when groups are large, if too many people are trying to contribute at once or, alternatively, if shyness is inhibiting several students.

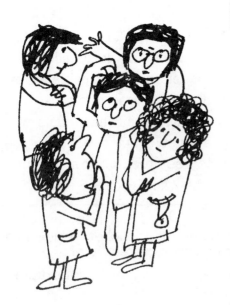

FIGURE 3·6
CONDUCTING A BUZZ
GROUP

FIGURE 3·7
CONDUCTING A BRAIN-
STORMING SESSION

Procedure

➡ the group is divided into sub-groups of 3–4 students

➡ discussion occurs for a few minutes (the term 'buzz' comes from the hive of verbal activity!)

➡ a clear task must be set

➡ each group reports back to the whole group

---

3. Brainstorming

This is a technique that you should consider when you wish to encourage wide and creative thinking about a problem. It is also valuable when highly critical group members (including perhaps yourself?) appear to be inhibiting discussion. If used frequently, it trains students to think up ideas before they are dismissed or criticized. The key to successful brainstorming is to separate the generation of ideas, or possible solutions to a problem, from the evaluation of these ideas or solutions.

Procedure

★ explain the rules of brainstorming to the group:

  ● criticism is ruled out during the idea generation stage

  ● **all** ideas are welcome

  ● quantity of ideas is the aim (so as to improve the chances of good ideas coming up)

  ● combination and improvement of ideas is sought

★ state the problem to the group

★ a period of silent thought is allowed during which students write down their ideas

★ ideas are then recorded (in a round robin format) on a blackboard, overhead transparency or butcher's paper for all to see

★ when **all** ideas are listed, and combination and improvement of ideas are complete, discussion and evaluation commences.

---

4. Role playing

This is a powerful and underused technique. It is very valuable in teaching interpersonal and communication skills, particularly in areas with a high emotional content. It has been found to be helpful in changing perceptions and in developing empathy. It is not a technique to use without some experience so you should arrange to sit in on a role play session before using it in your own course. In this regard, your colleagues teaching psychiatry or counselling should be able to help.

Procedure

- explain the nature and purpose of the exercise
- define the setting and situation
- select students to act out roles
- provide players with a realistic description of the role or even a script. Allow time for them to prepare and, if necessary, practice
- specify observational tasks for non-players
- allow sufficient time for the role play
- discuss and explore the experience with players and observers

5. Plenary session

In many group teaching situations, and indeed at medical conferences, subgroups must report back to the larger group. This reporting back can be tedious and often involves only the subgroup leaders who may present a very distorted view of what transpired. The plenary session method may help you get round these problems.

Procedure

- subgroups sit together facing other subgroups
- the chairman of subgroup A briefly reports the substance of the discussion in his group
- the chairman of subgroup B then invites members of subgroups B, C, D etc. to ask questions of any member of group A
- after 10 minutes chairman B reports on the discussion in subgroup B and the process is repeated for each subgroup
- the 10 minute (or other) time limit must be adhered to strictly.

6. Evaluation discussion

From time to time during a course it is desirable to review the progress of your small group, both in regard to the teaching and in regard to the material you are covering. There are a number of ways you could collect information about these matters, one of which is the technique called the evaluation discussion.

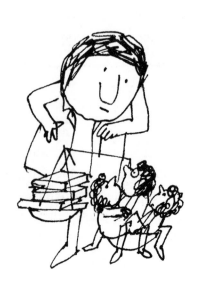

Procedure

 prior to the group meeting students are asked to write a 1-2 page evaluation of the group's work focussing equally on their reactions to the processes of teaching and what they are learning.

 each student reads this evaluation to the group

 each member of the group is then free to ask questions, agree or disagree, or comment

For success you must be sure to create an atmosphere of acceptance where negative as well as positive information can be freely given.

EVALUATING SMALL GROUP TEACHING

Evaluation implies collecting information about your teaching and then making judgements based on that information. Making judgements based on what one student says, or on rumour or intuition, is simply not good enough. You must collect information in a way that is likely to lead to valid judgements. However, constant evaluation of small group activities is not recommended as it may inhibit the development and working of the group. Evaluation may be of two types: informal or formal.

Informal evaluation: this can proceed from your careful reflection of what happened during your time with the group. You may do this by considering a number of criteria which you feel are important. For example, you may be interested in the distribution of discussion among group members, the quality of contribution, the amount of your own talk, whether the purpose of the session was achieved and so on. Of course, your reflections will be biased and it is wise to seek confirmation by questioning students from time to time. However, the importance of informal evaluations lies in your commitment to turn these reflections into improvements. If you are concerned with your own performance, the assistance of a trusted and experienced colleague sitting in on the group, or even just a discussion of your own feelings about the group, may be very helpful.

FIGURE 3·11

EXAMPLE OF TUTORIAL QUESTIONNAIRE (ADVISORY CENTRE FOR UNIVERSITY EDUCATION, UNIVERSITY OF ADELAIDE)

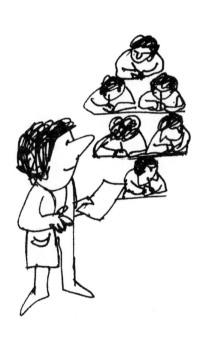

Name.............................. Course.................................

Please indicate your thoughts about the tutorial given by this particular tutor. Your responses are anonymous.

Indicate your present thoughts by means of a tick on the four-point scale.

(A) **The tutor**

good group leader	----	poor group leader
fits into the group	----	too forceful
likes opinions questioned	----	discourages the questioning of opinions
patient	----	impatient
sarcastic	----	never sarcastic
lively	----	monotonous
pleasant manner	----	unpleasant manner
interested in students	----	not interested in students
interested in my ideas	----	not interested in my ideas
interested in me as an individual	----	does not know me
encourages me to discuss problems	----	unable to discuss problems
treats me as an equal	----	treats me as a subordinate
clearly audible	----	mumbles
stresses important material	----	all material seems the same
makes good use of examples and illustrations	----	never gives examples
explanations clear and understandable	----	quite incomprehensible
appears confident	----	not confident

(B) **The tutorials**

well organized	----	muddled
good progression	----	poor progression
well prepared	----	not well prepared
time well spent	----	a waste of time
new material covered	----	merely repeat lecture material
have thrown new light on lecture course	----	irrelevant to understanding of lecture course
overcome difficulties encountered in lectures	----	difficulties not dealt with

(C) **The student's response**

I am fully aware of my progress	----	I seem to be 'working in the dark'
I enjoy contributing	----	I try to say nothing
I look forward to the tutorials	----	I would prefer not to attend
I have learnt a lot	----	I have learnt nothing
I am more inclined to continue with the subject	----	I have developed an aversion to the subject

Advice or suggestions for the future should be written on the back.

Formal evaluation: one formal approach to evaluation has already been described, the evaluation discussion. Other approaches include the use of questionnaires and the analysis of video recordings of the group at work. Standard questionnaires are available which seek student responses to a set number of questions. An example is shown in Figure 3.11.

Although such standard questionnaires can be useful you may find it more beneficial to design one that contributes more directly to answering questions which relate to your own course and concerns. As questionnaire design is a tricky business it is recommended that you seek the assistance of a teaching unit. The analysis of videotapes of your group at work is also a task which would require the expertise of someone from a teaching unit.

GUIDED READING

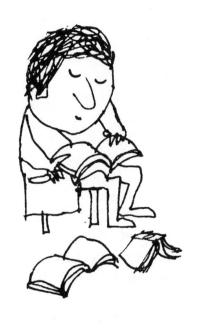

For a wide ranging discussion of the purposes and techniques of small group teaching we suggest you turn to M. L. J. Abercrombie's *Aims and Techniques of Group Teaching,* Society for Research into Higher Education (fourth edition), Guildford, Surrey, 1979. This monograph also provides a good introduction to the research literature on small groups.

If you are looking for a brief, practical guide to the use of discussion in small groups, you might find it helpful to obtain a copy of W.F. Hill's *Learning Thru Discussion,* Sage, Beverley Hills, California, 1982. The outlines in this book will help you get started if you are new to small group teaching. You will, of course, need to adapt some of the strategies to the circumstances of your own teaching.

Another excellent guide, to both the theory and the practice of group work, is D. Jacques, *Learning in Groups.* Croom-Helm, London, 1984.

Books and journals referred to in this chapter:

Experiences in Groups by W.R. Bion, Tavistock, London, 1968

Medical Humanities – A New Medical Adventure by A.R. Moore, New England Journal of Medicine, **295**, 1976, 1479–80

Learning Through Discussion at the Open University by A. Northedge, Teaching at a Distance, 2, 1975, 10–17

4: TEACHING PRACTICAL AND CLINICAL SKILLS

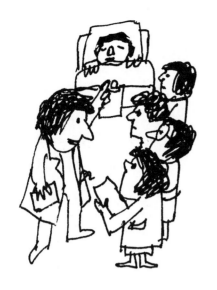

INTRODUCTION

In this chapter we plan to look at ways of improving your clinical teaching. It is unlikely that you will be able to obtain specific help in this matter as training courses in clinical teaching appear to be non-existent. It is a fact that clinical teaching is the most neglected of all areas of teaching. It is equally a fact that it is the area in which more deficiencies have been found than in any other. The conclusion of one extensive study was that 'many (clinical) teaching sessions, particularly ward rounds, were haphazard, mediocre and lacking in intellectual excitement'. In one study of medical schools in North America, it was stated that there were few students who could report having been monitored in the interview and physical examination of more than one or two patients and that a surprising number had been awarded their degree without ever having been properly supervised in the complete data-collecting process of even one patient! It is our experience, with notable exceptions, that a similar situation can be found in most medical schools in many other parts of the world.

THE ATTRIBUTES OF AN EFFECTIVE CLINICAL TEACHER

These have been identified on the basis of the opinions of experts, the perceptions of students and from the observations of actual clinical teaching. Considering the limited nature of the research there is a remarkable consistency in the results. It might be helpful to start by checking yourself against these attributes.

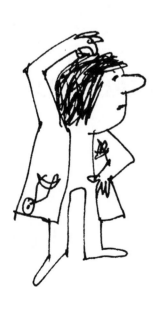

★ Do you encourage active participation by the students and avoid having them stand around in an observational capacity?

★ Do you have and demonstrate a positive attitude to your teaching?

★ Is the emphasis of your teaching on applied problem solving?

★ Do you focus on the integration of clinical medicine with the basic and clinical sciences or do you spend most of the time on didactic teaching of factual material?

★ Do you closely supervise the students as they interview and examine patients at the bedside and provide effective feedback on their performance or do you rely on their verbal case presentations in the teaching room?

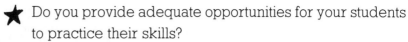

★ Do you provide adequate opportunities for your students to practice their skills?

★ Do you provide a good role model, particularly in the area of interpersonal relationships with your patients?

★ Does your teaching provide stimulation and challenge?

★ Is your teaching generally patient orientated or does it tend to be disease orientated?

★ Are you friendly, helpful and available to your students?

Should your honest answer to most of these questions be 'no' then you are probably a typical clinical teacher as many studies have shown that these attributes are rarely present. Just becoming aware of these attributes should encourage you to be more critical of your approach. The remainder of this chapter will deal more specifically with the planning and the techniques which can be introduced to enhance the effectiveness of your clinical teaching.

IMPROVING WARD-BASED TEACHING

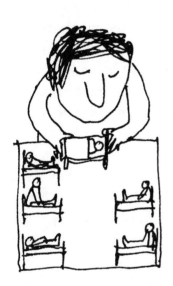

If you are a clinical teacher, with no responsibilities for the planning of the curriculum, there may be few educational initiatives open to you other than to improve your ward-based teaching. What you should aim to do is to try and acquire as many as possible of the attributes described in the previous section. There are no hard and fast rules as to how you can achieve this aim but the following points may be helpful.

Plan the teaching: it is unlikely that you will have received highly specific instructions from the Faculty unless you are teaching in a structured programme (see later). However, it is worthwhile contacting the Department Head or the Dean to see if there are defined objectives for the part of the curriculum in which your teaching is placed.

If these are not forthcoming, you should draw up your own objectives, at least to the extent of writing down what you hope to achieve during the students' attachment. In doing so you must take into account your time, the duration of the students' attachment, the number of the students and the seniority of the students. You must be realistic about what you can achieve and not attempt to cram too much into your sessions. You should inform the students about your plan and listen to any comments they may make which might reasonably give you cause to modify the plan. Though clinical teaching is essentially opportunistic, being dependent on the availability of patients, it is wise to keep a record of the conditions seen during your teaching so that by the end of the course you have covered a wide enough range of illustrative cases. You should, of course, co-ordinate your teaching with other tutors who are involved with your group of students.

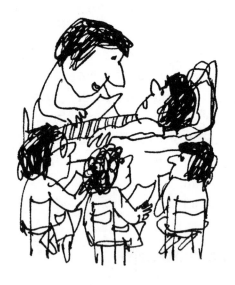

Set a good example: It is surprising how infrequently students get the chance to watch an experienced clinician take a history, perform an examination and subsequently discuss the outcome and plans with the patient. It is normally impossible for a consultant to do this on the working ward round because pressure of time means that decision making is given priority. However, the outpatient department often provides a better opportunity.

One of the difficulties students might have under such circumstances is the contrast between what you do in practice and what you expect of the students and this issue may have to be discussed. The important thing is for the students to see you in action, particularly in regard to the way you relate to the patients while at the same time achieve the medical aims of the encounter. Even on ward rounds it is important to demonstrate a concern for the patient's feelings.

Involve the student: The need for active participation is a recurrent theme throughout this book and nowhere is it more important than on the ward. You should take every opportunity to ask students to perform. This may range from talking to a patient, checking physical signs, presenting the case history, answering questions on the ward round and looking up clinical information for presentation at the next teaching session. In general try and make sure all the tasks are directly related to the patients currently on the ward. The emphasis of the teaching should, as Professor Andrew has put it, be 'bedside not backside'.

Observe the student: As mentioned earlier, a consistent finding in studies of clinical teaching has been a lack of direct observation of student interactions with patients. All too often the clinical teacher starts with the case presentation and may never check to see whether the features described are actually present or were elicited personally by the student. Serious deficiencies in clinical skills are consistently found in interns and residents which must be an indictment of the undergraduate clinical teaching. Only a commitment to the somewhat boring task of observing the student take the history, perform the physical examination and explain things to the patient will allow you to identify and correct any deficiencies. This type of activity is particularly essential with junior students and must be conducted in a sympathetic and supportive way.

Provide a good teaching environment: The more senior and prestigious you are, the more intimidating you are likely to appear to the students. It is vital that you adopt a friendly and helpful manner and reduce the natural and inevitable apprehensions felt by your students. Not only may they be apprehensive about you, but they will also be apprehensive about their impending contact with patients. You can assist this by preparing the patients and by showing to the students you understand their fears. Such fears are likely to be particularly evident with junior students.

IMPROVING THE CLINICAL TUTORIAL

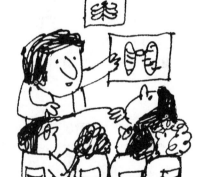

Clinical tutorials, even those conducted on the ward, are all too often didactic with the emphasis being on a disease rather than on the solving of patient problems. We firmly believe the clinical teacher should concentrate on the latter. The students will inevitably have many other opportunities to acquire factual information but relatively little time to grapple with the more difficult task of learning to apply their knowledge to patient problems. It is sad, but true, that in traditional medical schools the students are often as much to blame as their teachers by encouraging didactic presentations, particularly when examinations are imminent.

Plan the teaching: Once again it is important to establish the aims of the sessions you have been allocated. There may be fixed topics to cover or you may have a free hand. In either case you must be sure in your own mind what you intend to achieve in each session.

Involve the student: Make it clear from the beginning that you expect most of the talking to be done by the students and that all of them are to participate, not just the vocal minority. At the first session explain what tasks you expect them to perform in preparation for each tutorial. You may, for example, expect them to prepare cases for discussion or to read up aspects of the literature on a particular subject.

Provide a good teaching environment: The way in which you set up the session is vital for its success, particularly when you wish to encourage active participation. Your role as a facilitator, not the fount of all knowledge, must be emphasized and you must resist the temptation to jump in with extra information all the time. This is very hard to avoid but if it happens too frequently you will soon find all conversation is channelled in your direction and there will be no interaction between the students.

As the clinical tutorial is another form of small group teaching you should read the chapter on this subject for further advice.

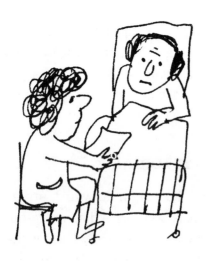

Concentrate on clinical problem solving: In the last twenty years there has been a substantial research effort into how doctors and students go about solving clinical problems. The findings have major implications for the clinical teacher, though as yet there is little evidence that this has been widely recognized. The traditional way of teaching students is to require them to take a full history, perform a comprehensive examination and then come up with a differential diagnosis. This logical and sequential approach has been shown to be fallacious. This is not the way doctors or students actually operate intellectually, even though they may appear to do so on superficial observation.

The work of Elstein, Barrows and others has shown that clinicians will generate diagnostic hypotheses with a minute or so of first seeing the patient. The bulk of time spent interviewing and examining the patient will then be used to confirm or refute these hypotheses. This approach to problem solving is a natural ability and does not have to be taught in its own right. However, successful clinical problem solving is dependent on experience and on effective utilization of the medical knowledge relevant to the problem. These findings explain why some new medical schools have used problem-based learning as the keystone of their curricula. They use patient problems to trigger the search for factual information rather than teaching factual information before exposing students to patient problems.

How to teach clinical problem solving: From what we have said the aim must be to provide your students with as much experience as possible in manipulating their factual knowledge in relationship to patient problems. You should avoid conducting tutorials in which you or your students present topics. If for example you wish to have a tutorial dealing with hypertension then a patient with hypertension should be the focus. The student can then be forced to consider the implications of hypertension in relation to that particular patient. Figure 4.1 briefly shows a plan for the simplest type of problem solving tutorial. There are many variations on the theme which you could introduce once you gain a little more experience.

FIGURE 4.1
A PLAN FOR A PROBLEM-
SOLVING TUTORIAL

Procedure

- a week before the tutorial, designate one or two students to prepare a case for presentation. Tell them they are to be prepared on all clinical and theoretical aspects of the case.

- at the start of the tutorial outline the aims of the exercise.

- get the prepared students to give the presenting complaint or allow the patient to tell the story.

- stop, and ask the other students what they think the problem or diagnosis could be. Ask them to justify their suggestions. Encourage the other students to react to these suggestions.

- allow the presentation of more data.

- stop again, and ask the group whether they have changed their views and why.

- continue the process.

This general approach is used not just for data gathering but also for the ordering of investigations (what tests would you order and why?) and treatment (what treatment would you give and why?). Though this may sound rather structured and formal, in practice this will not be so. You will soon learn to judge the pace, learn how much new information is to be given before stopping and so on. However, you may initially find sessions of this type hard going if the students are not used to the challenge of this method of teaching. Those previously relying on the regurgitation of lists and pages from the books may be particularly discomforted. They may attempt to avoid answering or justifying their suggestions but persistence will pay off.

With sessions of this type it is important to create a non-threatening atmosphere. One way of helping things along is to participate yourself. Let the presenting students bring along a case or patient whom you do not know. Still encourage the students to answer first but you can then add your own thoughts. You may even find this more threatening than the students but it is important they learn that infallibility is not an attribute of clinical teachers and that it is quite normal for even the most experienced clinician to have to admit indecision and a need to obtain advice or further information.

ALTERNATIVES TO TRADITIONAL WARD TEACHING

We have already provided evidence that traditional ward teaching is often inadequate in meeting the aims of both the Faculty and the students. This has led many schools to introduce structured courses to teach basic clinical skills in a less haphazard manner. The skills taught are often not restricted to interviewing and physical examination but include technical skills and clinical problem solving. Should you have the opportunity to introduce such an approach then the first step must be to define the objectives of the exercise. These must take into account the seniority of the students, the time available in the curriculum, the facilities, the availability of teachers and other resources.

There are obviously many ways in which this could be done but we will restrict ourselves to outlining such a programme that has been operating with success in our own school for over 10 years. It is one which has retained the support of both staff and students. This course was introduced in the fifth year of our six year curriculum because it became apparent that the unstructured ward-based teaching in the third and fourth years had left gaps in most students' basic skills.

The outline of the programme is shown in Figure 4.2. In the lefthand column you can see the objectives. Opposite each are the teaching activities which are planned to help the student achieve the objectives. In the righthand column are the assessment procedures which are also matched to the objectives. You can see that a wide range of methods are used. The key to the programme is the attachment of only three students to a preceptor for instruction on history taking and physical examination. You will note that the problem orientated medical record approach has been adopted and we find this a very valuable adjunct to our teaching. Whole group problem-solving sessions include clinical decision

FIGURE 4.2

COURSE PLAN FOR A
STRUCTURED COURSE ON
BASIC CLINICAL SKILLS

OBJECTIVES	TEACHING ACTIVITIES	ASSESSMENT
TAKE A COMPREHENSIVE HISTORY	PRECEPTOR SESSIONS WITH VIDEOTAPE RECORDINGS. WARD ACTIVITIES.	PRECEPTOR'S JUDGMENT BASED ON VIDEOTAPE RECORDING AT END OF COURSE
PERFORM A COMPLETE PHYSICAL EXAMINATION	VIEWING DEMONSTRATION VIDEOTAPE. PRECEPTOR SESSIONS. WARD PRACTICE. WARD ROUNDS WITH REGISTRARS	PRECEPTOR JUDGMENT. OBSERVATION OF COMPLETE PHYSICAL EXAMINATION BY INDEPENDENT EXAMINER AT END OF COURSE.
WRITE-UP HISTORY AND EXAMINATION AND CONSTRUCT A PROBLEM LIST	PROBLEM-ORIENTED CASE WRITE-UPS ON WARD PATIENTS. PRECEPTOR SESSIONS	CASE WRITE-UPS
DECISIONS ON DIAGNOSIS, INVESTIGATIONS AND MANAGEMENT	WHOLE-GROUP PROBLEM-SOLVING SESSIONS. CASE WRITE-UPS	WHOLE GROUP TUTOR'S OPINION. CASE WRITE-UPS
ABILITY TO RELATE TO PATIENTS	PRECEPTOR SESSIONS WITH REVIEW OF VIDEOTAPE RECORDINGS.	PRECEPTOR'S JUDGMENT
IMPROVE KNOWLEDGE OF MEDICINE AND SURGERY	SELF-INSTRUCTION. PREPARATION OF CASES FOR PRESENTATION TO THE WHOLE GROUP. COMPUTERIZED SELF-ASSESSMENT PROGRAMMES. TAPE-SLIDE TUTORIALS	WHOLE GROUP TUTOR'S OPINION. SELF-ASSESSMENT

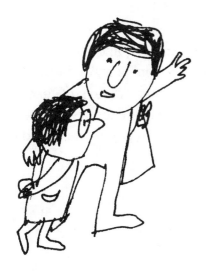

making, emergency care, data interpretation (clinical chemistry, haematology and imaging) and management-therapeutics. The students are also expected to take responsibility for a lot of their own learning.

As it has been decided that the time of the teaching staff should be devoted to preceptoring and conducting small group sessions, the revision of the theoretical aspects of medicine and surgery is left entirely to the students. Various self-instructional programmes (e.g. tape-slide presentations, computerized self-assessment modules) are also available for the students to undertake in their own time.

Though such a programme is far from perfect, it was introduced within a traditional curriculum and with the minimum of resources. The main change was a re-allocation of staff time away from didactic activities and into more direct observation of student performance.

A perusal of the medical educational literature will provide you with many other examples of structured clinical teaching. From the Netherlands, you will find the concept of a 'clinical skills laboratory' where medical schools have set up fully staffed and equipped areas devoted to putting groups of students through an intensive training in clinical skills, often using a wide range of simulations.

From America you will find descriptions of several courses designed to tackle the difficult area of training in interpersonal skills and counselling. All have the same general approach: to undertake the training of various clinical skills in a structured and supervised way to ensure that all students achieve a basic level of competence.

TECHNIQUES FOR TEACHING PARTICULAR PRACTICAL AND CLINICAL SKILLS

Many practical and clinical skills can be taught as separate elements. Because there are many of these elements, and as ward-based teaching is generally haphazard, many medical schools have established programmes to teach basic skills in a piecemeal fashion. This is normally done early in the students' career, often just prior to their first clinical attachments. Much of this has come about because of new technology (e.g. video recording, computers) and because of an awareness of the value of simulation in its many forms. This section will introduce you to a variety of ways of teaching basic skills some of which may not be of immediate relevance but some of which ought to be in operation in your medical school because of their proven efficacy.

The clinical interview

There are two basic methods with which you ought to be familiar: the use of video recordings and the use of simulation.

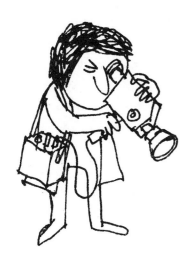

Video recording: Any department which has the responsibility for teaching aspects of history taking or interpersonal skills should have access to video recording equipment, preferably of the portable kind that can be set up in ward side rooms, outpatients and other teaching areas. You should become familiar with the technical operation of the equipment, a skill which is often now taught to primary school children so should not be beyond the capacity of the average medical teacher.

There are several ways in which video equipment can be used. The simplest is to record examples of interviewing techniques (good and bad) for demonstration purposes. This may be valuable as a starting point for new students. You may also wish to have an example of a basic general history so the novice student can get an idea of the questions that are routinely asked. Some medical schools have recorded segments of interviews with patients which show various emotional reactions (e.g. aggressive behaviour, grief, manipulation).

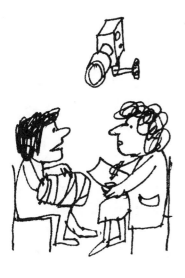

The most powerful way of using the video is to record the student's interview with a patient. This may be initially stressful but both student and patient usually forget they are being recorded after a few minutes. A time limit of 20–30 minutes is advisable. The student, or a small group of students, meet later with the teacher to review the tape. It is at this stage that some skill by the teacher is required. Firstly, the situation must be a supportive one to allow frank and open discussion. Secondly, the teacher must have a clear idea of what he intends to teach. (If you have not read formally in the area of the clinical interview, we would recommend the books by Enelow and Swisher and by Morgan and Engel.)

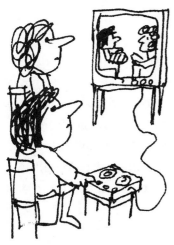

It is not appropriate to play the tape completely through and then have a discussion. The tape must be stopped frequently to discuss points as they arise. Such things as non-verbal cues, aspects of doctor–patient relationships, avoidance of jargon, adequacy of questions, direction of the enquiry, directive versus non-directive questioning, hypothesis generation and many other issues can be identified and discussed, both with the interviewing student and with the student's peers. Such sessions are valuable both with junior and senior students.

There are clearly several advantages of this approach over direct observation. The teacher is not committed to be present at the actual interview, the teaching can be scheduled at a convenient time, a recorded interview can be interrupted as often as necessary and most importantly the student can review his own performance. The latter by itself often produces a striking impact and a rapid improvement in performance.

Simulation: The use of simulated patients is another well proven and powerful method for teaching interview skills. However, it does require some expertise to train the simulated patients and if you wish to pursue this technique we strongly recommend that you read the book by Barrows. The simulated patient offers certain distinct advantages over the real patient particularly for the novice student. The analogy has been drawn with the value of flight deck simulators in pilot training. The advantages include the ability to schedule interviews at a convenient time and place, all students can be faced with the same situation, the interview can be interrupted and any problems discussed freely in front of the 'patient', there is no risk of offending or harming the patient (often a concern of new students), the student can take as much time as necessary, the same 'patient' can be re-interviewed at a later date and the simulator can be trained to provide direct feedback, particularly in the area of doctor-patient relationships.

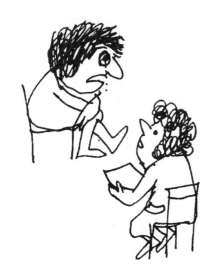

Simulations can also be developed for situations that are usually impossible for students to experience with real patients. This is particularly so for emotionally charged areas.

With all these advantages it is surprising how little this technique is used. Much is due to uninformed prejudice. Some is due to a lack of appreciation as to how easy it is to train simulated patients. This is not an appropriate place to deal with this aspect in depth. However, it is important to remember that simulated patients need not necessarily be actors. Indeed, our preference is to avoid actors, who may wish to give a performance rather than to be a 'patient'. The basic technique is to identify a patient with the condition you wish to simulate. A protocol is drawn up of the facts which are relevant to that condition. All other aspects of this history not relevant to the condition need not be simulated, i.e. the simulator's own background can be used or adapted. The simulator then learns the role, including non-verbal cues. The trainer then tests the simulation by taking the history. Modifications are made and further practice sessions conducted. It is then our practice to try out the simulation by 'admitting' the simulator to the ward and asking one of the resident staff to conduct an interview. This is observed and a discussion held with the resident about the patient. It is readily apparent whether the resident suspects the simulator of not being real. It is, in fact, very rare for a well trained simulator to be suspected, which is a good confidence booster for both the simulator and trainer.

The physical examination

Video recording: Video recordings can be used to help students develop physical examination skills in much the same way as for interviewing skills. However, it is not quite so effective and direct observation and instruction are generally more appropriate. It is very valuable to have videotapes which illustrate the recommended way of performing specific components of the examination. These must be readily available to students together with playback facilities convenient to the wards.

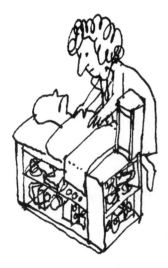

Simulation devices: This is the area where technology has made a major contribution. These devices include those for cardiac auscultation, breast examination, prostate palpation, pelvic examination and laryngeal examination.

Simulated patients: These can also be used in very much the same way as for history taking, with similar advantages. However, the range of signs that can be simulated is limited, though not as much as you might think. Barrows has shown that a very wide range of neurological conditions can be simulated.

In regard to other systems, conditions where pain is the main feature are particularly suitable. Also valuable are simulations of emergency situations such as perforation of a viscus, myocardial infarction and subarachnoid haemorrhage. Students can be trained to perform rapid assessment and acute management for conditions that otherwise would be impossible to programme.

Simulated patients are quite widely used in North America to teach the pelvic examination. The main advantage of such an approach is that the patient gives direct feedback on the students' performance. The patient is the only one who can say if the student has correctly palpated the ovaries and uterus or whether unnecessary discomfort has been created. The same approach has been used to teach rectal examinations in the male.

Though not simulation, it is perhaps worthwhile reminding you that self and peer examination is a valuable teaching technique for novice students. The learning of basic manual skills is much better done in this way than using real patients.

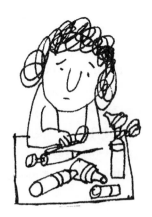

The use of instruments and basic equipment

The student has to become competent with a variety of instruments and basic medical equipment other than the stethoscope. These include the ophthalmoscope, the auroscope, the proctoscope, the laryngoscope, syringes, infusion apparatus, lumbar puncture needles, and endotracheal tubes. For many of these, simulation devices are available. In most cases it is unfair if the first attempt to use them is made on a patient. Students will certainly appreciate the chance to practice their skills in a situation where they are not going to hurt a patient.

Some techniques, of course, are readily practiced on each other (e.g. examinations of the eyes, ears and throat).

EVALUATING CLINICAL AND PRACTICAL TEACHING

There are few well-developed procedures for evaluation in these areas of teaching. You can, of course, adapt the principles and procedures described previously (p. 16; p. 50) and integrate these with the checklist displayed at the very beginning of this chapter.

You may have gained the impression that we favour the use of questionnaires in evaluation. We wish to point out that this is not the case. Questionnaires are only **one** method which seek data from **one** source – typically your students. In all evaluation, including clinical and practical teaching, we would wish to encourage you to explore other methods and other sources of evaluative information. Consult the section of evaluation at the end of Chapter 5 for some ideas on these methods.

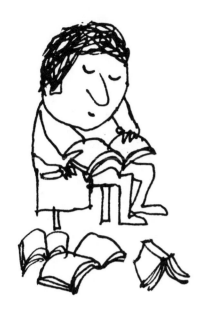

GUIDED READING

Although there are many good books written on how to perform a medical interview and a physical examination, there seems to be a dearth of books on clinical teaching. There is, of course, a substantial journal literature on the subject. Should you wish to read further, we refer you to the following two review articles:

The Art and Science of Clinical Teaching, A.M. Yonke, *Medical Education,* **13**, 1979: 86–90.

Research on Clinical Teaching by C.J. Daggett, J.M. Cassie, and G.F. Collins, *Review of Educational Research,* **49**, 1979: 151–169

Clinical Teaching Strategies for Physicians by P.J. McLeod and R.M. Harden, *Medical Teacher* **7**, 1985, 173–189.

Books and articles referred to in this chapter:

The Clinical Approach to the Patient by W.L. Morgan and G.L. Engel, W.B. Saunders, Philadelphia, 1969.

Interviewing and Patient Care by A.J. Enelow and S.N. Swisher, Oxford University Press, New York, 1972.

Simulated Patients (Programmed Patients) by H.S. Barrows, Charles C. Thomas, Springfield, Illinois, 1971.

Medical Problem Solving: An Analysis of Clinical Reasoning by A. Elstein, L. Shulman and S. Sprafka, Harvard University Press, Cambridge, Massachusetts, 1978.

Reflections on Clinical Teaching and Learning by R.R. Andrew, Australian Family Physician, 6, 1977: 1053–1057.

5: PLANNING A COURSE

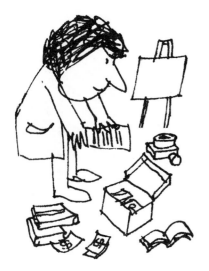

INTRODUCTION

This chapter aims to assist you when you become involved in some way in planning a course and wish to do so in a systematic manner. Unfortunately, there is no straightforward formula to guide you in this activity. The reasons for this are twofold. Firstly, course design is a complex business involving more than purely educational considerations. For example, you will find that full account must be taken of the context in which you teach. Lucky is the planner who can rely on the full co-operation of the teaching staff, has an adequate budget and does not have to take account of departmental or faculty politics. Secondly, relatively few courses are started from scratch. Most course design work is a matter of revising and redesigning existing courses.

In our view, the key to good course design is to forge educationally sound and logical links between intentions (objectives), teaching and learning methods and the assessment of student learning. Too many courses start with vague intentions, consist of teaching which has a tenuous relationship to these intentions and employ methods of assessment which bear little or no relationship to either. They then place students in the unfortunate situation of playing a guessing game, with their academic future as the stake! This pattern can only be improved by adopting a systematic approach which links the intentions with the teaching and the assessment.

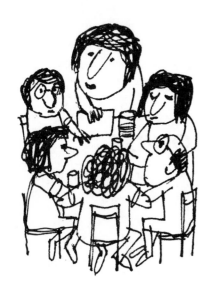

WHO SHOULD BE RESPONSIBLE FOR COURSE DESIGN?

Although this chapter assumes you have some responsibility for course design it is unlikely that this will be a solo affair. You have additional resources on which to draw which may include staff of your own and related departments, staff of a university teaching unit with experience in course design work, members of the profession outside your immediate environment and students. These people may form a planning committee or a panel of advisers. Whatever your situation, experience suggests that some form of consultation with others is necessary to avoid planning errors.

OBJECTIVES AND COURSE DESIGN

The intentions of the course are usually expressed in the form of **learning objectives.** Objectives are clear statements of what students should be able to do as a result of a course of study. They must be carefully distinguished from **aims** which are usually statements of what a teacher intends to do and from **goals** which indicate what a course or perhaps an institution is seeking to achieve. We are convinced that clear statements of objectives are a fundamental tool in course design because they make the rational choice of teaching and learning activities possible and are essential in planning a valid assessment of student learning. Unfortunately, many teachers seem to have an antipathy to thinking about, let alone writing, objectives. However, a course designer without objectives is proverbially 'up the creek without a paddle'. The relationship between objectives, teaching and learning activities, and assessment is best set out in a **course planning chart** such as that seen in Figure 5.1.

FIGURE 5·1
EXAMPLE OF A COURSE PLANNING CHART

OBJECTIVES	TEACHING AND LEARNING ACTIVITIES	ASSESSMENTS
AT THE COMPLETION OF THE COURSE THE STUDENT WILL BE ABLE TO:		
1 TAKE A COMPREHENSIVE HISTORY	1 PRECEPTOR SESSIONS WITH REVIEW OF VIDEO RECORDINGS OF PATIENT INTERVIEWS	1 PRECEPTOR'S JUDGMENT BASED ON VIDEO RECORDING OF A HISTORY AT THE END OF COURSE
2	2	2
3	3	3

Each defined objective is matched with appropriate teaching and learning activities and with a valid form of assessment. For instance, in the example above, you would not expect the students to learn to be able to 'take a comprehensive history at the completion of the course' on the basis of lectures, nor would you expect that this could be validly assessed by a paper-and-pencil test. The course designer has provided a relevant teaching and learning activity and a more suitable form of assessment.

WRITING OBJECTIVES

Before you start writing objectives it might help to know what they should look like. Here are some simple examples:

★ Identify benign and malignant skin lesions.
★ Understand environmental factors that predispose young children to disease.
★ Obtain a problem-orientated history from a patient.
★ Perform a venepuncture.
★ Demonstrate a willingness to be critically evaluated by peers.

In each case, the objective contains an **operative** word (such as identify or obtain) which indicates the kind of behaviour that students will be required to demonstrate in order to show that the objective has been achieved. Now, if you look at each objective again, you will notice that they suggest rather different kinds of behaviour. The first two objectives require information of an intellectual kind for their achievement and may be classified as **knowledge objectives**. The third and fourth objectives refer to a skill of a practical kind and are thus **skill objectives.** The last objective suggests an attitude of mind and is therefore classified as an **attitudinal objective.**

These three broad divisions are often used in grouping objectives but you will certainly come across several refinements of each division in the literature. The most common of these is the taxonomy developed by Bloom and his colleagues. They call the three divisions **domains:** cognitive (knowledge and intellectual skills), psychomotor (physical skills) and affective (feelings and attitudes). These domains have been subdivided to provide hierarchies of objectives of increasing complexity.

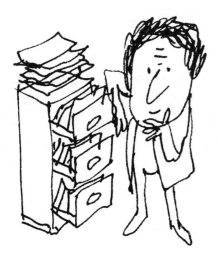

Knowledge objectives (the cognitive domain): It is in this area that Bloom's taxonomy has been most widely applied. He proposes six levels – knowledge, comprehension, application, analysis, synthesis and evaluation. Though these provide an intellectual framework for considering objectives, for everyday use you may find it more practical to 'collapse' them into three more general subdivisions:

- Recall of information
- Understanding
- Problem solving

The reason for keeping these different levels in mind when writing objectives is that courses frequently pay undue attention to one level (usually the recall of information).

Skill objectives (the psychomotor domain): Bloom and his colleagues did not develop a hierarchy of objectives in the psychomotor domain, though others have attempted to do so. The medical teacher will need to pay a great deal of attention to developing skill objectives. Such objectives can be improved if the conditions under which the performance is to occur and the criteria of acceptable performance are indicated. Conditions of performance may specify whether the student is to be working with real or simulated patients, the kind of data they will be given to assist in diagnosis and so on. The standard of performance may be a simple statement such as 'without error' or 'in accordance with the checklist'.

Another way you might find useful is to specify competent performance using the hierarchy developed by Korst. He suggests that in any area of medicine there will be some skills with which one would expect students to show a high degree of competence and others with which one might only expect familiarity (Figure 5.2).

FIGURE 5.2
SKILL OBJECTIVES
(AFTER KORST)

STANDARD OF PERFORMANCE	EXAMPLE OF SKILLS
WELL QUALIFIED OR VERY COMPETENT	• CARDIAC RESUSCITATION • BLOOD PRESSURE DETERMINATION • VENOUS PULSES IN NECK • ARTERIAL PULSES IN ARMS, LEGS AND NECK
FAMILIAR WITH OR COMPETENT	• INTERPRETATION OF CHEST X-RAY • FUNDAL EXAMINATION IN HYPERTENSION
AWARENES OR MINIMAL FAMILIARITY	• CARDIAC CATHETERIZATION • CORONARY ARTERIOGRAPHY • PERICARDIOCENTESIS

Our own final year objectives for Medicine and Surgery are written in a similar way (Figure 5.3).

FIGURE 5.3
EXAMPLE OF SKILL
OBJECTIVES (UNIVERSITY
OF ADELAIDE)

A GIVEN APPROPRIATE EQUIPMENT THE STUDENT SHOULD BE ABLE TO PERFORM THE TASKS AND PROCEDURES LISTED BELOW

1 URINALYSIS
2 STOOL EXAMINATION FOR OCCULT BLOOD
3 THORACOCENTESIS
4 OPTHALMOSCOPY
5 ETC.

B THE STUDENTS SHOULD HAVE OBSERVED THE FOLLOWING PROCEDURES

1 ENDOSCOPY (UPPER G.I.)
2 PLEURAL BIOPSY
3 LIVER BIOPSY
4 JOINT ASPIRATION
5 ETC.

C THE STUDENT SHOULD BE ABLE TO INTERPRET THE FOLLOWING INVESTIGATIONS

1 COMMON ECG ABNORMALITIES
2 ARTERIAL BLOOD GAS REPORTS
3 ROUTINE PULMONARY FUNCTION REPORTS
4 COMMON X-RAY ABNORMALITIES
5 ETC.

Attitudinal objectives (the affective domain): Writing objectives in the affective area is very difficult, which possibly explains why they are so often ignored. This is unfortunate because, implicitly or explicitly, there are many attitudinal qualities we hope to have in our graduating students. As Krathwohl has a taxonomy in this domain you could approach the task in much the same way as writing knowledge objectives.

Another way is to attempt to define the starting attitudes of the students and match these with more desirable attitudes towards which you would hope they would move. For example, you could be concerned with the attitude of students to other health professionals. You might start by assuming that the students had a stereo-typed image of the role of other health professionals. You would then wish to move them **away from** this **towards** an attitude which demonstrated respect and acceptance of the place of other health professionals. The advantage of this method is that it recognizes that not all students will achieve the desired attitude nor will they all necessarily start a course with the same attitudes.

Where do objectives come from?

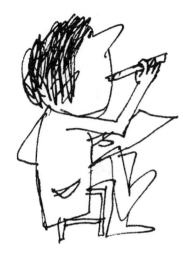

Writing objectives is not simply a process of sitting, pen in hand, waiting for inspiration, although original thinking is certainly encouraged. Objectives will come from a consideration of the subject matter, what you and your colleagues know about the subject, and what is being taught. This may not be so easy if you have to design a course from scratch. In this case you should consider a wide range of sources for objectives. These include:

- your own knowledge, skills and attitudes
- your colleagues' knowledge, skills and attitudes
- practitioners' knowledge, skills and attitudes
- students' interests
- the knowledge, skills and attitudes of students as they enter the course
- information in the literature
- patient and community health needs
- the objectives of the department or faculty
- published taxonomies and lists of objectives from other courses and institutions.

How specific and detailed should objectives be?

This is a question frequently asked. The answer depends on the purposes for which the objectives are to be used. In designing a course, the objectives will be more general than the objectives for a particular teaching session within the course. As objective writing can become tedious and time consuming it is best to keep your objectives simple, unambiguous and broad enough to clearly convey your intentions. The objectives for a six week clinical skills course, conducted for groups of 9–10 fifth year students, is shown below. Though quite broad, these objectives have proved detailed enough for course planning purposes and for making the intentions of the programme clear to students.

FIGURE 5·4
EXAMPLE OF COURSE
OBJECTIVES

OBJECTIVES	TEACHING AND LEARNING ACTIVITIES	ASSESSMENTS
AT THE COMPLETION OF THE COURSE THE STUDENT WILL BE ABLE TO		
1 TAKE A COMPREHENSIVE HISTORY	1	1
2 PERFORM A COMPLETE PHYSICAL EXAMINATION	2	2
3 WRITE UP THE HISTORY AND EXAMINATION AND CONSTRUCT A PROBLEM LIST	3	3
4 MAKE DECISIONS ON DIAGNOSIS, INVESTIGATION AND MANAGEMENT	4	4
5 RELATE WELL TO PATIENTS	5	5
6 SHOW THAT HE/SHE HAS IMPROVED HIS/HER KNOWLEDGE OF MEDICINE AND SURGERY	6	6

RELATING OBJECTIVES TO TEACHING AND LEARNING ACTIVITIES

One of the main purposes in producing a clear set of objectives is to help you to select **appropriate** teaching and learning activities. By appropriate we mean activities that enable the objectives to be achieved and that are feasible in your own particular circumstances. Clearly, it would be inappropriate to plan to use computer-assisted instruction, however desirable this method might be, if your teaching department had no access to computing facilities or there was no one prepared or able to produce effective computer-assisted instructional materials.

The main types of **teaching** undertaken in medical schools, such as lecturing, small group teaching and clinical teaching, are dealt with in earlier chapters. These are by no means all of the methods available with other possibilities including practical classes, peer teaching and a variety of simulation techniques. In addition, it should be remembered that students undertake many **learning** activities in the absence of teaching. This should be kept in mind with due allowances being made for **independent** learning. It is not unreasonable to make explicit in your objectives, areas where you expect the students to work on their own. This particularly applies to knowledge objectives which might be achieved just as well independently as by a series of didactic lectures. It could also apply to skill objectives where students might be expected to seek out clinical and practical experience by themselves.

The way in which this process has been followed through in our fifth year clinical skills course is demonstrated once again on the course planning chart (Figure 5.5). When planning this

FIGURE 5·5

EXAMPLE OF MATCHING TEACHING AND LEARNING ACTIVITIES TO COURSE OBJECTIVES

OBJECTIVES	TEACHING AND LEARNING ACTIVITIES	ASSESSMENTS
AT THE COMPLETION OF THE COURSE THE STUDENT WILL BE ABLE TO 1 TAKE A COMPREHENSIVE HISTORY	1 PRECEPTOR SESSIONS WITH REVIEW OF VIDEO RECORDINGS OF PATIENT INTERVIEWS	
2 PERFORM A COMPLETE PHYSICAL EXAMINATION	2 VIEWING DEMONSTRATION VIDEOTAPE. PRECEPTOR SESSIONS WITH PATIENTS. WARD PRACTICE. WARD ROUNDS WITH RESIDENT STAFF	
3 WRITE UP THE HISTORY AND EXAMINATION AND CONSTRUCT A PROBLEM LIST	3 TAPE-SLIDE PROGRAMME ON PROBLEM-ORIENTED RECORD KEEPING. WRITE-UPS ON WARD PATIENTS. PRECEPTOR SESSIONS TO CHECK AND DISCUSS WRITE-UPS.	
4 MAKE DECISIONS ON DIAGNOSIS, INVESTIGATIONS AND MANAGEMENT	4 PROBLEM-BASED WHOLE GROUP DISCUSSION SESSIONS. REVIEW OF CASE WRITE-UPS.	
5 RELATE WELL TO PATIENTS	5 PRECEPTOR SESSIONS WITH REVIEW OF VIDEO RECORDINGS OF PATIENT INTERVIEWS.	
6 SHOW THAT HE/SHE HAS IMPROVED HIS/HER KNOWLEDGE OF MEDICINE AND SURGERY	6 INDEPENDENT LEARNING. PREPARATION OF CASES FOR PRESENTATION. TAPE-SLIDE TUTORIALS. COMPUTERIZED SELF-ASSESSMENT PROGRAMMES.	

course we were aware that many students were deficient in their basic history taking and physical examination skills. We thus decided to put the majority of our staff time into achieving the first two objectives. The most appropriate teaching method was obviously direct observation and as this is very time consuming we opted for a preceptor system where one staff member was responsible for only three students throughout the programme. However, opportunity was also provided for students to obtain additional ward practice on their own and the resident staff were also mobilized to provide additional help and instruction in this area. One of the implications of this decision on staff allocation was to accept that the sixth objective (Improving their knowledge in the subjects Medicine and Surgery) would have to be achieved by other methods. This has involved an expectation that students accept responsibility for doing much of this themselves. We have also designed and prepared a variety of self-instructional materials. Other teaching techniques are incorporated to achieve other objectives.

RELATING OBJECTIVES TO ASSESSMENT METHODS

In the same way as it is important to match the teaching and learning methods with the objectives, it is equally important to match the assessment methods to the objectives. Failure to do so is an important reason why courses fail to live up to expectations. A mismatch of assessment and objectives may lead to serious distortions of student learning (see also Chapters 6 and 8).

In designing your course, we believe it is important to distinguish carefully between two types of assessment. One is primarily designed to give feedback to the students as they go along (**formative assessment**). The other is to assess their abilities for the purposes of grading (**summative assessment**). Formative assessment is a crucial part of the educational process, especially where complex skills are to be mastered. Such assessment is notoriously deficient in medical schools, particularly in regard to clinical teaching.

The way in which assessment was designed into our fifth year clinical skills course is shown in Figure 5.6. As no formal examination is required at the completion of the course the major emphasis of the assessment activities is formative. However, assessment activities of a summative type are conducted during the final two weeks of the programme when aspects of the student's performance are observed by preceptors and by other staff members. You will note that the assessment of knowledge is left largely to the students themselves. In other circumstances we might have used a written test to assess this component of the course.

FIGURE 5·6

EXAMPLE OF MATCHING ASSESSMENT PROCEDURES TO COURSE OBJECTIVES

OBJECTIVES	TEACHING AND LEARNING ACTIVITIES	ASSESSMENTS
AT THE COMPLETION OF THE COURSE THE STUDENT WILL BE ABLE TO 1 TAKE A COMPREHENSIVE HISTORY	1 PRECEPTOR SESSIONS WITH REVIEW OF VIDEO RECORDINGS OF PATIENT INTERVIEWS.	1 ASSESSMENT OF VIDEO RECORDING DURING COURSE (FORMATIVE). ASSESSMENT OF VIDEO RECORDING AT END OF COURSE (SUMMATIVE).
2 PERFORM A COMPLETE PHYSICAL EXAMINATION	2 VIEWING DEMONSTRATION VIDEO TAPE. PRECEPTOR SESSIONS WITH PATIENTS. WARD PRACTICE. WARD ROUNDS WITH RESIDENT STAFF.	2 DIRECT OBSERVATION DURING COURSE (FORMATIVE). DIRECT OBSERVATION AT END OF COURSE (SUMMATIVE).
3 WRITE UP THE HISTORY AND EXAMINATION AND CONSTRUCT A PROBLEM LIST	3 TAPE-SLIDE PROGRAMME ON PROBLEM ORIENTATED RECORD KEEPING. WRITE-UPS ON WARD PATIENTS. PRECEPTOR SESSIONS TO CHECK AND DISCUSS WRITE-UPS.	3 MARKING AND DISCUSSION OF CASE WRITE-UPS DURING COURSE (FORMATIVE). MARKING OF CASE WRITE-UPS AT END OF COURSE (SUMMATIVE).
4 MAKE DECISIONS ON DIAGNOSIS INVESTIGATION AND MANAGEMENT	4 PROBLEM-BASED WHOLE GROUP DISCUSSION SESSIONS. REVIEW OF CASE WRITE-UPS.	4 PERFORMANCE IN WHOLE GROUP SESSIONS (SUMMATIVE).
5 RELATE WELL TO PATIENTS	5 PRECEPTOR SESSIONS WITH REVIEW OF VIDEO-RECORDINGS OF PATIENT INTERVIEWS.	5 ASSESSMENT OF VIDEO RECORDINGS DURING COURSE (FORMATIVE AND SUMMATIVE).
6 SHOW THAT HE/SHE HAS IMPROVED HIS/HER KNOWLEDGE OF MEDICINE AND SURGERY	6 INDEPENDENT LEARNING. PREPARATION OF CASES FOR PRESENTATION. TAPE/SLIDE TUTORIALS. COMPUTERIZED SELF-ASSESSMENT PROGRAMMES.	6 SELF-ASSESSMENT. COMPUTERIZED SELF-ASSESSMENT PROGRAMMES (FORMATIVE).

SEQUENCING AND ORGANIZING THE COURSE

It is unlikely that the way in which you have set out your objectives, teaching and assessment on the planning chart will be the best chronological or practical way to present the course to students. There are several things that must be done. Firstly there must be a **grouping** of related objectives and activities. (In the example we are following throughout this chapter, such a grouping occurs for objectives one to three which are largely to be achieved by the preceptor sessions.) Secondly, there must be a **sequencing** of the teaching activities. There are likely to be circumstances in our own context that influence you to sequence a course in a particular way, such as hospital routines or university teaching terms. However, there are also a number of educational grounds upon which to base the sequencing. These include:

* the logical or historical development of a subject
* important themes or concepts
* proceeding from what students know to what they do not know
* proceeding from concrete experiences to abstract reasoning
* starting from unusual, novel or complex situations and working backwards towards understanding.

TRADITIONAL VERSUS INNOVATIVE CURRICULA

The approach to course design we have presented is particularly relevant to the teacher working within the context of a traditional medical school. However, it is important to be aware of new approaches to medical education, lessons from which may become pertinent even to the most conventional institution. These so-called innovative schools have developed concepts which are variably referred to as 'problem-based', 'student-centred', 'community-based'. The emphasis tends to be on facing students with clinical problems at an early stage in the curriculum as a prelude and stimulus to the learning of the relevant basic and clinical science. The students are usually expected to undertake much of the learning on their own and in small groups. Lectures tend to be at a minimum with staff resources being used more to facilitate group activities. A good review of the differences between traditional and innovative curricula can be found in an article by Harden and his colleagues.

OTHER COURSE DESIGN CONSIDERATIONS

Many of the important educational considerations in designing a course have been addressed, but there are other matters that must be dealt with before a course can be mounted. These are only briefly described because the way in which they are handled depends very much on the administrative arrangements of the particular situation in which you teach. Having said that, we are not suggesting in any way that your educational plans must be subservient to administrative considerations. Clearly, in the best of all possible worlds, the administrative considerations would be entirely subservient to the educational plans but the reality is that there will be a series of trade-offs, with educational considerations hopefully paramount.

In planning your new course, you will need to take the following into account.

Administrative responsibilities: Unless you are working alone, it will be necessary for one person to assume the responsibility of course co-ordination. This job will require the scheduling of teachers, students, teaching activities, assessment time and resources.

Allocation of time: Many courses are over ambitious and require far more time (often on the part of students) for their completion than is reasonable. This is especially true if it is part of a larger course of study. In allocating time, you will need to consider the total time available and its breakdown, and how time is to be spent in the course. It is often desirable to use blocks of time to deal with a particular topic, rather than 'spinning it out' over a term or a year.

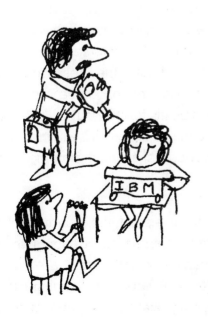

Allocation of teaching rooms, clinics, laboratories and equipment: Courses depend for their success on the careful allocation of resources. Allocative procedures vary, but it is important that all competing claims are settled early in a departmental meeting so that orderly teaching can take place.

Technical and administrative support: Whether you teach a course alone, or as one of a team, you will find a need for support of some kind or other. It may be as simple as the services of a typist to prepare course notes and examination papers, or as complex as requiring, at different times, the assistance of audio-visual technicians to help prepare materials, theatre staff, laboratory staff and computer programmers. Your needs for support must be considered at the planning stage.

EVALUATING THE COURSE

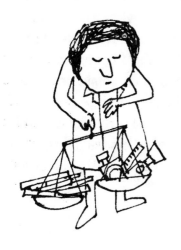

Many teachers may find a discussion of course evaluation in a chapter on design rather odd, perhaps believing that this activity is something that takes place **after** a course has been completed. We believe this generally should not be the case. It is our contention that in teaching you should be progressively evaluating what you are doing and how the course design and plans are working out in practice. In this way, modifications and adjustments can be made in a planned and informed manner. But what is evaluation? You will often find the terms 'evaluation' and 'assessment' used interchangeably, but evaluation is generally understood to refer to the process of obtaining information about a course (or teaching) for subsequent judgement and decision making. This process, properly done, will involve you in rather more than handing around a student questionnaire during the last lecture. What you do clearly depends on what you want to find out, but thorough course planning and course revision will require information about three different aspects of your course. These are the context of and inputs into your course, the processes of teaching, learning, assessment and course administration and, finally, the outcomes of the course.

Context and input evaluation: This is crucial if mistakes and problems are not to be sheeted home, unfairly, to teachers. In this type of evaluation you will need to consider the course in relation to such matters as other related courses, the entering abilities and attitudes of students, the resources and equipment available to teach with and, of course, the overall design and planning arrangements for the course. The major sources of information you can use here will be in the form of course documents, student records, financial statements and the like.

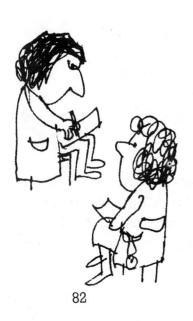

Process evaluation: This focusses on the conduct of the teaching, learning, assessment and administration. It is here that the views of students can be sought as they are the only people who experience the full impact of teaching in the course. Questionnaires, written statements, interviews and discussion are techniques that you can consider.

Outcome evaluation: This looks at student attainments at the end of the course. Naturally you will review the results of assessment here and judge whether they meet with the implied and expressed hopes for the course. Discussion with students and observation of aspects of their behaviour will help you determine their attitudes to the course you have taught.

In all evaluations, whether it is evaluation of a course or evaluation of teaching, it is helpful to keep in mind that there are many sources of information available to you and a variety of methods you can use (Figure 5.7).

FIGURE 5.7
COURSE/TEACHING
EVALUATION

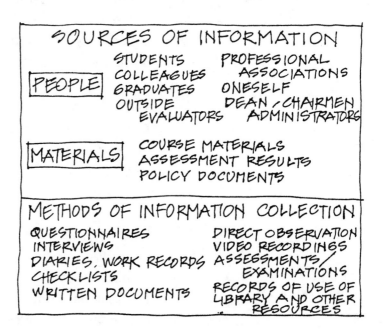

The literature on evaluation will guide you on using these diverse sources and methods. We recommend the reference to Roe and McDonald in the knowledge that it contains many helpful practical examples of checklists, interview schedules and questionnaires. You may also wish to refer to the course evaluation questionnaire at the end of Chapter 1.

GUIDED READING

For a useful extension of the material in this chapter we suggest you have a look at the appropriate sections in Beard and Hartley's book *Teaching and Learning in Higher Education*, Harper and Row, London, 1984.

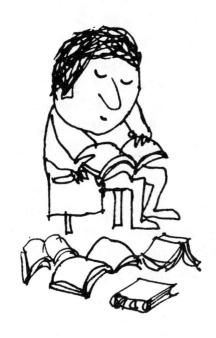

If you are keen to look at course planning in depth, you could obtain a copy of the book by D. Dallas *et al.* entitled **Studies in Course Design,** Volume 1, University Teaching Methods Unit (now the Centre for Staff Development in Higher Education), University of London, 1978.

Another helpful textbook on course planning has been written by William H. Berquist, *et al.* Entitled **Designing Undergraduate Education**, it examines the following six curricular dimensions: time, space, resources, organization, procedures and outcomes. This book was published by Jossey-Bass, San Francisco, in 1981.

The literature on objectives is very extensive. A useful guide is the book by R. Beard, F.G. Healey and P.J. Holloway called **Objectives in Higher Education** (second edition), Society for Research in Higher Education, London, 1974.

The self-instructional book by R. Mager, **Preparing Instructional Objectives**, (second edition) Lake, Belmont, California, 1984 is a useful how-to-do-it guide by one of the most well known advocates of the use of objectives in teaching.

For a thorough discussion of evaluation, plus examples of evaluation methods (e.g. questionnaires), we suggest you obtain a copy of: E. Roe and R. McDonald, **Informed Professional Judgement: A Guide to Evaluation in Post-secondary Education**. University of Queensland Press, Brisbane, 1983.

Books and articles referred to in this chapter:

Taxonomy of Educational Objectives. Handbook I: Cognitive Domain by B.S. Bloom *et al.,* McKay, New York, 1956.

Taxonomy of Educational Objectives. Handbook II:Affective Domain by D.R. Krathwohl, B.S. Bloom and B.B. Masia, McKay, New York. 1962.

A Guide to the Clinical Clerkship in Medicine by D.R. Korst, University of Wisconsin, 1973.

Educational Strategies in Curriculum Development: the SPICES Model by R.M. Harden, S. Sowden and W.R. Dunn. *Medical Education,* **18**, 1984, 284–297.

6: ASSESSING THE STUDENTS

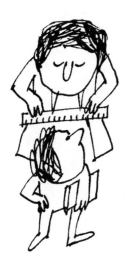

INTRODUCTION

Being involved in student assessment is perhaps the most critical of all tasks facing the teacher. Generally, teachers take such involvement quite seriously but, sadly, the quality of many assessment and examination procedures leave much to be desired. The aim of this chapter, therefore, will be to help you to ensure that the assessments with which you are involved will measure what they are supposed to measure in as fair and as accurate a way as possible. We will provide some background information about the purposes of assessment and the basic principles of educational measurement. We will then detail the forms of assessment with which you should be familiar in order that you can rationally select the best method to use.

THE PURPOSE OF THE ASSESSMENT

When faced with developing an assessment you must be quite clear about its purpose. This may appear to be stating the obvious but try asking your colleagues what they think is the purpose of the assessment with which you are concerned. We are certain that there will be a considerable diversity of opinion. Some may see it as testing the students' mastery of the course content, others may see it as a way of ranking the students, and yet others as a way of encouraging students to study the course vis-à-vis another concurrent course.

Mehrens and Lehmann identify several purposes of assessment which may be paraphrased as follows:

- Judging mastery of essential skills and knowledge.
- Measuring improvement over time.
- Ranking students.
- Diagnosing student difficulties.
- Evaluating the teaching methods.
- Evaluating the effectiveness of the course.
- Motivating students to study.

Though it may be possible for one assessment method to achieve more than one of these purposes, all too often assessments are used for inappropriate purposes and consequently fail to provide valid and reliable data.

It must never be forgotten how powerfully an assessment affects students, particularly if it is one on which their future may depend. This influence may be a positive one or a negative one and even a harmful one. For many students, passing the examination at the end of the course is their primary motivation. Should this examination not be valid, and thus not truly reflect the content and objectives of the course, then the potential for serious distortions in learning and for making errors of judgement about students is evident. An example from our own experience may illustrate this point. A revision of the final year curriculum inadvertently led to the multiple-choice test component of the end of year assessment having considerably more weight than the clinical component. Students were observed to be spending excessive amounts of time studying the theoretical aspects of the course in preference to practising their clinical skills, the latter being the main aim of the curriculum revision. A subsequent modification of the assessment scheme, giving equal weighting to an assessment of clinical competence, has corrected this unsatisfactory state of affairs.

It is our view that assessments on which decisions about the students' future are to be made (summative assessment) should be kept quite separate from assessments which are for the benefit of the students in terms of guiding their further study (formative assessment).

Summative assessment

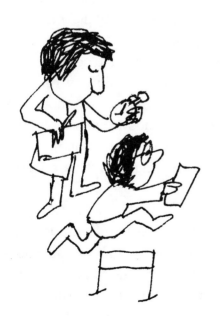

In dealing with summative assessment, every effort must be made to ensure that all tests are good tests so that any decisions made are fair and based on the appropriate criteria. Students should be fully informed of these criteria, on the test methods to be employed and on the weightings given to each component. Such information should preferably be given to students when a course begins. This is important because it is surprising how often information obtained from other sources, such as past students or even from the department itself, can be inaccurate, misleading or misinterpreted by the students. The best way of avoiding this is to provide printed details of the course plan, including the assessment scheme. Examples of past papers can be provided and we have found an open forum on the assessment scheme early in the course to be both popular and valuable.

Formative assessment

Formative assessments can be organized more informally. Such assessments must be free of threat as the aim is to get the students to reveal their weaknesses rather than to disguise them and, equally importantly, to allow them to demonstrate their strengths. Opportunities to obtain feedback on knowledge or performance are always appreciated by students and lead to positive feelings about the department and the staff concerned.

WHAT YOU SHOULD KNOW ABOUT EDUCATIONAL MEASUREMENT

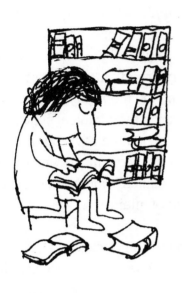

Whatever the purpose of the assessment, the method used should satisfy the following three requirements:

1. **Validity:** Does it measure what it is supposed to measure?
2. **Reliability:** Does it produce consistent results?
3. **Practicability:** Is it practical in terms of time and resources?

For example, a test of blood sugar would be invalid if it actually measured blood alcohol. It would be unreliable if the sample of blood gave different results on repeated analyses. It would be impracticable if it took two technicians three hours to perform at a cost of $500 per test. This simple example may appear to insult your intelligence but analogous education examples of invalid and unreliable tests can be found in most, if not all, medical schools. For instance, the results of multiple-choice examinations are frequently used as a major component of examinations which are used to certify clinical competence. Though such tests may be high on reliability they are predictably low on validity. Another example is the traditional clinical viva which continues to be widely used despite the evidence showing the performance of the examiners to be so inconsistent as to make such assessments very unreliable.

Our intention in raising these matters is to encourage you to apply the same critical interest in the quality of educational tests as you undoubtedly apply to those tests you use in your research or in the investigation of your patients. This section will provide you with some basic information about aspects of educational measurement with which we think you should be familiar.

Validity

Content validity is the first priority of any assessment. It is a measure of the degree to which it contains a representative sample of the knowledge and skills it was meant to cover. A numerical value cannot be placed against it and it must be subjectively judged according to the objectives of the assessment. Therefore in approaching any assessment the first question you must ask is: **what are the objectives?**

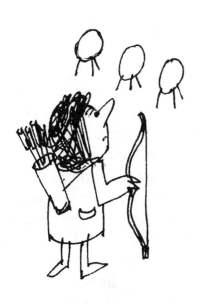

Unfortunately, in many medical schools such objectives are not available, either for the institution or for individual courses. Should you be in this situation, with no written objectives for the assessment you have to design, then you have no alternative but to develop your own. This is not such a difficult task as you might imagine because, as far as the assessment is concerned, the objectives are embodied in the course content. A look at the teaching programme, lecture and tutorial topics, and discussions with teaching staff should allow you to identify and categorize the key features of the course. What you are, in fact, attempting to do is to construct a course plan in reverse and you may find it helpful at this point to consult the chapter on course design where this process is discussed in greater detail.

The objectives of the course, however categorized, are the framework against which you can evaluate the content validity. For the content validity to be high, the assessment must sample the students abilities **on each objective**. As these objectives are likely to cover a wide range of knowledge, skills and attitudes, it will immediately become apparent that no single test method is likely to provide a valid assessment. (For instance, a multiple-choice test will hardly be likely to provide valid information about manipulative skills.) This sounds simpler in theory than it actually is in practice. Some objectives, particularly those in the attitudinal area, will be hard to assess in an examination setting. In such cases, alternative forms of assessment should be sought. For example, you might have to agree that the attitudinal objectives of the course should come from supervisors' ratings despite the problems you anticipate with their reliability.

There are two other forms of validity known as **construct validity** and **criterion-related validity**. Generally speaking you will not be in a position to evaluate these aspects of validity so we will not discuss them further.

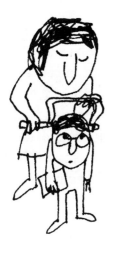

Reliability

The reliability of any assessment is a measure of the consistency and precision with which it tests what it is supposed to test. Though its importance is initially less vital than validity, you should remember that an unreliable assessment cannot be valid. The degree of reliability varies both with the test format itself and with the quality of its application.

Theoretically, a reliable test should produce the same result if administered to the same student on two separate occasions. The statistic describing the degree to which this happens is called the coefficient of stability. In most situations, practical considerations make it impossible to provide such information. This difficulty is normally overcome by providing a measure of **internal consistency**. The basic principle of this statistical technique is to split the test into two parts and assume they are equivalent. A test with a high degree of internal consistency shows a high correlation between the student's performance on each half of the test. The most commonly used statistics of this type are the Kuder–Richardson formulae. You will frequently come across them in computer scored multiple-choice tests.

The other key component in determining the reliability of a test is the **consistency of the marking**. This factor is responsible for the unacceptable levels of reliability in most forms of direct assessment, in clinical examinations and in written tests of the essay type. However, methods are available to help you minimize this problem and will be discussed later in this chapter.

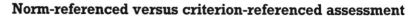

Norm-referenced versus criterion-referenced assessment

Before we finish dealing with some of the basic principles of educational measurement we wish to be satisfied that you understand the difference between norm and criterion-referenced assessment. You are likely to be familiar with norm-referenced assessment as this reflects the traditional approach to testing. Any assessment which uses the results of all the students to determine the standard is of this type. In such tests the pass level is often determined arbitrarily, by pre-determining the proportion of students given each grade or statistically, by using the standard deviation.

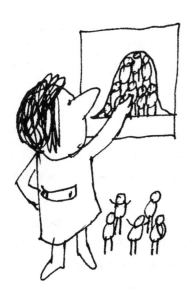

In the professional field we should be more concerned that the students achieve some minimal standard of competence. If this is the main purpose of the assessment then the criterion-referenced approach is the more appropriate. Such an approach necessitates the determination of the standard before the examination is conducted rather than waiting to see the overall results before doing so. Though this is extremely difficult to do, and even then often has to be modified for practical reasons (e.g. too many students would fail), we have found that attempting to do so is a powerful way of improving the validity of the assessment. Everyone concerned is forced to consider each item in the examination and ask themselves if it is relevant and set at the appropriate level of difficulty. Our own experiences with such an examination used to test clinical competence in the final year have been very rewarding.

ASSESSMENT METHODS

In planning your assessment, it is clearly necessary to be aware of the variety of methods available to you. It is impossible to be comprehensive for reasons of space so we will restrict ourselves to those methods most commonly in use in medical schools. We will also include information about some of the more innovative approaches which have been developed recently which may be of interest. We do this deliberately in an attempt to encourage you to become subversive. With your new found knowledge of assessment you will soon be involved in situations where it is obvious that inappropriate methods are being used. This may be due to a combination of tradition, ignorance or prejudice. The first two you may be able to influence by rational argument based on the type of information we provide in this book. The latter is a more difficult problem with which to deal.

TYPES OF ASSESSMENT

1 Essay
2 Short-answer
3 Structured (written)
4 Objective (multiple choice, true-false)
5 Direct observation
6 Oral
7 Structured (practical/clinical)

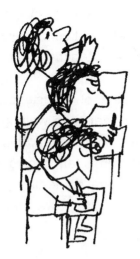

1. ESSAY

Essay tests have become quite rare in medical school assessments for several reasons. Though they are relatively easy to set they are extremely time-consuming to mark. The widespread use of multiple-choice tests and the advent of computer scoring has lifted the marking burden from many academics, few of whom would wish to take it up again. Excluding such selfish reasons, there are also other reasons for avoiding essays, the most important being the potential for unreliable marking. Several studies have shown significant differences between the marks allocated by different examiners and even by the same examiner remarking the same papers at a later date.

All in all, we recommend caution in the use of an essay test except in situations where its unique attributes are required. The essay is the only means we have to assess the students ability to compose an answer and present it in effective prose. It can also indirectly measure attitudes, values and opinions.

Essay questions tend to be of two kinds. The first is the **extended response** kind. An example is seen in Figure 6.1.

FIGURE 6.1
EXAMPLE OF EXTENDED
RESPONSE ESSAY
QUESTION

> DESCRIBE WHAT SERVICES YOU THINK SHOULD BE PROVIDED BY A COMMUNITY HEALTH CENTRE. GIVE REASONS FOR YOUR SELECTION OF SERVICES AND PROVIDE ILLUSTRATIONS FROM CENTRES OPERATING IN AT LEAST TWO DIFFERENT REGIONS

In the extended response question the student's factual knowledge, ability to provide and organize ideas, to substantiate them and to present them in coherent English are tested. The extended essay is useful for testing knowledge objectives at the higher cognitive levels.

Another type of essay question is the **restricted response** kind, an example of which is shown in Figure 6.2.

FIGURE 6.2
EXAMPLE OF RESTRICTED
RESPONSE ESSAY
QUESTION

> KIDNEY DISEASE IS A SIGNIFICANT CAUSE OF HYPERTENSION
> DESCRIBE THE MECHANISM BY WHICH THIS OCCURS

This type of essay is best used for testing lower level knowledge objectives. An advantage of the more restricted format is that it decreases the scoring problems.

If you intend to set essay questions, then we suggest that you keep in mind the points in Figure 6.3.

FIGURE 6·3
PROCEDURE FOR SETTING
AND MARKING ESSAY
QUESTIONS

Procedure

 Write questions that elicit the type of response suggested by the objectives:
- Use clear directive words such as 'describe', 'compare', 'contrast', 'criticize' and 'explain'. If 'discuss' is used, be sure to indicate what points should be discussed.

- Establish a clear framework which aims the student to the desired response. Rather than: 'Discuss beta-blockers', try: 'Describe the benefits and potential hazards of beta-blockers in the treatment of heart disease'.

B **Set a relatively large number of questions requiring short answers of about a page rather than a few questions requiring long answers of three or more pages.**

This will provide a better sampling of course content and you will reduce bias in marking for quantity rather than quality.

C **Ensure that all students are required to answer the same questions:**

Constructing optional questions of equal difficulty is hard and, further, you will not be able to make valid comparisons among students if they have answered different questions.

D **Prepare a marking system:**

Two methods are commonly used, both of which require you to prepare a model answer. In the **analytical method** of marking, a checklist of specific points is prepared against which marks are allocated. Such factors as 'logical argument' or 'expression' should be included if you think they are relevant. If you wish to reward legibility and presentation give these components a proportion of the marks but avoid these aspects unduly biasing your assessment of the content. The **global method** of marking can be used if you have at least 30 papers to mark. Papers are read rapidly and assigned to one of five or more piles, grading from a superior response down to the inferior. Papers are then re-read to check the original sorting. This is a faster and more reliable method of marking once standards for the various piles have been established.

Mark questions with the following points in mind:
- Mark anonymously
- Mark only one question at a time or, preferably, have a separate marker for each question.
- Adopt consistent standards.
- Try to mark one question without interruption.
- Preferably have two independent markers for each question and average the result, or at least re-read a sample of papers to check marking consistency.

2. SHORT-ANSWER

Short-answer tests have been surprisingly little used in recent times; yet another casualty of the multiple-choice boom. Though short-answer questions require hand marking this should not produce major problems with reliability as long as well-constructed marking sheets are prepared. As such marking can be done quickly and efficiently any objections from teaching staff can be attributed to laziness! Short-answer questions can be sought from your colleagues in the same way as you might seek multiple-choice questions.

FIGURE 6.4
EXAMPLES OF SHORT-
ANSWER QUESTIONS
WITH ANSWER KEYS

AN ELDERLY PATIENT PRESENTS WITH A TREMOR WHICH IS PRESENT AT REST, MADE WORSE BY ANXIETY AND DECREASED WITH INTENTION. YOU NOTE THAT THIS IS NOT PRESENT WHEN THE PATIENT IS ASLEEP. WHAT IS THE LIKELY DIAGNOSIS

ANSWER PARKINSONISM (1 MARK)

A SERUM BIOCHEMICAL SCREEN REVEALS A LOW CALCIUM, A LOW PHOSPHATE AND A RAISED ALKALINE PHOSPHATASE. LIST TWO TYPICAL SYMPTOMS YOU WOULD EXPECT THIS PATIENT TO HAVE

ANSWER BONE PAIN; MUSCLE WEAKNESS; DIFFICULTY IN WALKING
(1 MARK FOR TWO CORRECT ANSWERS; ½ MARK FOR ONE CORRECT ANSWER)

Obviously more questions of this type can be fitted into a fixed time period than with essays. If one of the purposes of the assessment is to cover a wide content area then short-answer questions have distinct advantages. Much the same may be said about multiple-choice questions but short-answer questions have distinct advantages in that they avoid the use of cueing or the need for a single correct answer. In our experience, particularly in clinical subjects, it is possible to set an examination with a high level of content validity more easily with short-answer questions than with multiple-choice questions. The questions are easier to construct and you will be able to prepare questions to test areas you would find almost impossible to test using a multiple-choice format.

If you wish to employ short-answer questions you should take account of the points in Figure 6.5.

FIGURE 6.5

PROCEDURE FOR SETTING AND MARKING SHORT-ANSWER QUESTIONS

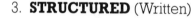

Procedure

A Make the questions precise.

B Prepare a structured marking sheet.
- Allocate marks or part marks for the acceptable answer(s).
- Be prepared to consider other equally acceptable answers, some of which you may not have predicted.

C Mark questions with the following points in mind:
- Mark anonymously.
- Complete the marking of one page of questions at a time.
- Preferably have a different examiner for each page of questions.

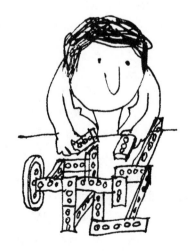

3. **STRUCTURED** (Written)

There are two types of structured tests with which we think you should be familiar. These are the **patient management problem** (PMP) and the **modified essay question** (MEQ). They are widely used by bodies constructing certifying examinations but less extensively used in medical schools, with notable exceptions. Both claim to assess problem solving skills.

Patient management problem

The typical PMP begins with a variable amount of patient data followed by a series of options from which the student can select (see Figure 6.6). Opposite each option is a box which contains instructions on how to proceed. These instructions are obscured by one of a variety of technical devices which include invisible ink, tabs and special paint which can be removed with an eraser. The instructions pass the student on to a data gathering section where selections are made from a wide range of possibilities. The student then proceeds sequentially through other sections dealing with diagnosis, investigation and management.

You are an intern working on a general medical unit of a teaching hospital. A man, aged 74, is admitted under your care. He presents with this letter from his general practitioner:

'Mr. Jones has been short of breath on exertion and complains of noises in his ears and no energy. He looks anaemic and his diet is probably inadequate. Please perform a blood picture and treat him if the anaemia is confirmed.'

You would NOW (select ONLY ONE of the following items and follow the directions given in the exposed response):

002	Ring the general practitioner	☐
003	Take a problem based history (suspected anaemia)	☐
004	Take a screening history (systems enquiry)	☐
005	Perform a screening examination	☐
006	Order immediate investigations	☐
007	Talk to the patient's relatives	☐
008	Ring your registrar	☐

These supposed simulations of clinical problem solving may employ a paper and pencil format as described or may utilize a computer, in which case rather more sophisticated formats can be introduced.

The PMP has several virtues. It has content validity and clearly measures skills not tested by most written tests. Though the proponents claim that it measures problem-solving skill, the relationship of performance on PMPs to performance in real life is far from clear. The methods of scoring have come under a lot of criticism. However, PMPs have their attractions and are popular with students. We find them to be particularly valuable for feedback where they generate much discussion about the pathways and decisions taken.

If you have not previously done so we suggest you obtain a PMP and have a go at it yourself. Should you then feel it would have value in your course you could obtain one of the books which shows you how to construct a PMP. You could expect it to take 20–40 hours of work to produce your first PMP.

Modified essay question

This test was initially developed for the Royal College of General Practitioners in London. The MEQ has not been extensively used but we believe the method deserves a wider application. The use of the term essay is perhaps a little misleading because the format more closely resembles a series of short-answer questions than an essay.

The student is provided with a limited amount of patient data, much as in the PMP, and then asked to write a brief answer to a question. Such questions may relate to history taking, examination findings, diagnosis, investigations and so on. Following one or more initial questions, further information is provided and additional questions are posed.

FIGURE 6·7

EXAMPLE OF THE START OF A MODIFIED ESSAY QUESTION

Please answer all the questions in sequence. Do **not** look through the book before you start.

Mr Smith, a 78 year old widower who lives alone, complains of lethargy and weight loss. He has been admitted to the general medical unit on which you work for further investigation.

Q1. What are the **three** most likely diagnoses?
a.
b.
c.

Q2. List **five** specific questions which would help you distinguish between these possibilities.
a.
b.
c.
d.
e.

A routine blood test ordered by his general practitioner reveals a haemoglobin of 10.4 g/dl and the anaemia is reported to be of the microcytic hypochromic type.

Q3. List **two** typical clinical signs you would look for when you examine the patient.
a.
b.

Q4. Briefly describe how this information has affected your first diagnosis.

A certain amount of skill is required when preparing an MEQ to avoid giving the answers to previous questions and to avoid the student being repeatedly penalized for the same error. Scoring is by comparison of the student's answer with model answers. The precautions to be taken in marking are the same as those described for marking short-answer questions.

MEQs are very popular with students, particularly when used in formative assessment. Marked papers can be returned or the students can be given the model answers and mark their own. The value of this exercise is enhanced when a tutorial is held to discuss disputes with the model answers. Should you wish to use this type of assessment then we recommend you start by obtaining a copy of the booklet listed in the guided reading.

4. OBJECTIVE TESTS

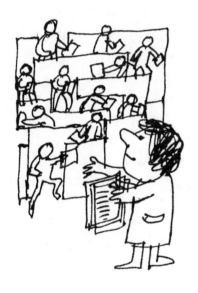

This generic term is used in education to include a variety of test formats in which the marking of the answers is objective. Some classifications include short-answer questions in this category. In medical education the term multiple-choice test is often used synonymously with the term objective test and, indeed, we have been guilty of doing so in early sections of this chapter. However, we encourage you to use this more general term as it allows us to include a wide variety of test types, only one of which can be described as 'multiple-choice'. Other commonly used examples of objective tests are the true-false and matching types.

The characteristics of such tests are the high reliability of the scoring, the rapidity of scoring and economy of staff time in this task, and the ability to screen large content areas. They lend themselves to the development of banks of questions, thus further reducing the time of examination preparation. These advantages have led to an over-reliance on objective tests and a failure to be critical in their use.

There is some debate on whether objective test items can be written to measure higher level intellectual skills such as problem solving. It may be that those very skilled in writing such items can do so but in one study there was little agreement among teachers and students with regard to the level of items in a surgical examination. When students were asked to verbalize the process by which they arrived at their answer it was shown that they usually arrived at correct answers at a low taxonomic level (recall and recognition) irrespective of the teacher's taxonomic classification of the item. Problem solving strategies were used by better students for answering any item for which the answer was not known. Though we do not wish to discourage you from attempting to write items which test more than the recall of factual information, we hope you will not delude yourself into believing that your objective tests measure more than they in fact do.

Whilst it is possible that you may never have to set or mark an essay test or a structured test, it is almost certain you will have to participate in some way in writing or administering multiple-choice tests. It is therefore your responsibility to have quite a detailed knowledge about this type of assessment. Though we will not be able to be comprehensive, we will attempt to provide you with enough information to do your job competently. This section will therefore contain more technical detail than the other sections in this chapter. We will have to leave it to your judgement as to how much of this detail is relevant to you.

Choosing the type of question

You must first find out or decide which type of item you will be using. Objective items, as we have said before, can be classified into three groups: **true-false, multiple-choice** and **matching**. Though much has been written about the advantages and disadvantages of each type, the differences are unlikely to exert any significant influence on the outcome of the assessment. We would suggest you stick to the true-false and multiple-choice types and avoid the more complex matching types which, in medical examinations, often seem to behave more like tests of IQ rather than tests of the course content. We also see little merit in using more than one item type within any single assessment.

True-false questions

Examples of true-false questions are shown in Figures 6.8 and 6.9.

FIGURE 6.8

EXAMPLE OF SIMPLE
TRUE - FALSE ITEM

FIGURE 6.9

EXAMPLE OF MULTIPLE
(CLUSTER) TRUE-FALSE
ITEM

(T) F   IN A 40-YEAR-OLD PATIENT WITH MILD HYPERTENSION YOU WOULD CONSIDER COMMENCING TREATMENT WITH PROPRANOLOL

IN A 40-YEAR-OLD PATIENT WITH MILD HYPERTENSION YOU WOULD CONSIDER COMMENCING TREATMENT WITH

- (T) F   PROPRANOLOL
- T (F)   HYDRALAZINE
- (T) F   BENDROFLUAZIDE
- T (F)   CLONIDINE
- T (F)   PRAZOSIN

The **simple type** will obviously cause you the least problems in construction and scoring. The more complex **multiple type** (also known as the cluster type) is very popular because it allows a series of questions to be asked relating to a single stem or topic. Some people have made life difficult by devising several ways of scoring this type. Each question may be marked as a separate question. However, the questions may also be considered as a group with full marks given only if all the questions are correct with part marks given if varying proportions of the questions are correct. Organizers of post-graduate examinations seem to be particularly partial to such variations. Research has shown that the ranking of students is unaltered by the marking scheme.

If you intend to use true-false questions you should take particular care of the following points:

FIGURE 6.10

PROCEDURE FOR SETTING
TRUE - FALSE QUESTIONS

Procedure

A Make sure the content of the question is important and relevant and that the standard is appropriate to the group being tested.

B Use statements which are short, unambiguous and contain only one idea.

C Ensure the statement is indeed unequivocally true or false.

D Avoid words which are giveaways to the correct answer, such as sometimes, always or never.

E Make sure true statements and false statements are the same length and are written in approximately equal numbers.

F Avoid negative or double negative statements.

100

Multiple-choice questions

An example of a simple multiple-choice question is shown in Figure 6.11.

FIGURE 6·11

EXAMPLE OF A SIMPLE
MULTIPLE- CHOICE ITEM

IN A 40-YEAR-OLD PATIENT WITH MILD HYPER-
TENSION WHICH ONE OF THE FOLLOWING WOULD
YOU USE TO COMMENCE TREATMENT?
1. PROPRANOLOL
2. HYDRALAZINE
3. CLONIDINE
4. PRAZOSIN
5. DIAZOXIDE

The MCQ illustrated is made up of a stem (In a 40-year...commence treatment?) and five alternative answers. Of these alternatives one is correct and the others are known as 'distractors'.

FIGURE 6·12

PROCEDURE FOR SETTING
MULTIPLE- CHOICE
QUESTIONS

Procedure

A Make sure the content of the question is important and relevant and that the standard is appropriate to the group being tested.

B The main content of the question should be in the stem and the alternatives should be kept as short as possible.

C Eliminate redundant information from the stem (this fault often applies to clinical items containing patient data).

D Ensure each distractor is a plausible answer which cannot be eliminated from consideration because it is irrelevant or silly.

E Avoid giving clues to correct or incorrect responses which have nothing to do with the content of the question.

- make sure correct and incorrect responses are of similar length;
- check the grammar, particularly when the alternative is written as the completion of a statement in the stem;
- distribute the place of the correct response equally among positions 1 to 5 (or 1 to 4 as the case may be).

F Do not use an 'all of the above' or 'none of the above' alternative.

G Avoid negatives.

H Do not try to write trick questions.

One advantage of the MCQ over the true-false question is a reduction in the influence of guessing. Obviously, in a simple true-false question there is a 50% chance of guessing the correct answer. In a one from five MCQ there is only a 20% chance of doing so if the distractors are working effectively. Unfortunately it is hard to achieve this ideal and exam-wise students may easily be able to eliminate one or two distractors and thus reduce the number of options from which they have to guess. Information about the effectiveness of the distractors is usually available after the examination if it has been computer marked (see section on item analysis).

If you intend to use multiple-choice questions you should take particular note of the points in Figure 6.12.

Context-dependent questions

Having mastered the basic principles of setting good objective items, you may wish to become more adventurous. It is possible to develop questions with a more complex stem which may require a degree of analysis before the answer is chosen. Such items are sometimes known as context-dependent questions. One or more multiple-choice questions are based on stimulus material which may be presented in the form of a diagram, graph, table of data, a statement from a text or research report, a photograph and so on. This approach is useful if one wishes to attempt to test the student's ability at a higher intellectual level than simple recognition and recall of factual information.

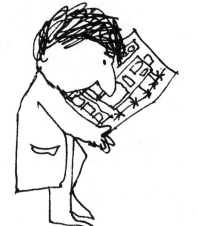

Putting together an objective test

This is the point where many tests come to grief. It is not enough to simply select a 100 items from a bank or from among those recently prepared by your colleagues. The selection must be done with great care and must be based on the objectives of the course. A blueprint should be prepared which identifies the key topics of the course which must be tested. The number of questions to be allocated to each topic should then be determined according to its relative importance. Once this is done the job becomes easier. Sort out the objective items into the topics and select those which cover as many areas within the topic as possible. It is advisable to have a small committee to help at this stage in order to check the quality of the questions and to avoid your personal bias in the selection process. You may find that there are some topics for which there is an inadequate number or variety of questions. You should then commission the writing of additional items from appropriate colleagues or if time is short, your committee may have to undertake this task.

The questions should now be put in order. It is less confusing to students if the items for each topic are kept together. Check to see that the position of the correct answers are randomly distributed throughout the paper and if not, re-order accordingly. Deliver the paper to the secretary for typing with suitable instructions about the format required and the need for security. At the same time make sure the 'instructions to students' section at the beginning of the paper is clear and accurate. Check and recheck the typed copy as errors are almost invariably discovered during the examination, a cause of much consternation. The use of a word processor would help considerably during this phase. Finally, take the paper to the printer and arrange for secure storage until the time of the examination.

Scoring an objective test

The main advantage of the objective type tests is the rapidity with which scoring can be done. This requires some attention to the manner in which the students are to answer the questions. It is not usually appropriate to have the students mark their answers on the paper itself. When large numbers are involved a separate structured sheet should be used. Where facilities are available it is convenient to use answer sheets that can be directly scored by a computer or marking machine. However, a hand marking answer sheet can easily be prepared. An overlay is produced by cutting out the positions of the correct responses. This can then be placed over the student's answer sheet and the number of correct responses are easily and rapidly counted.

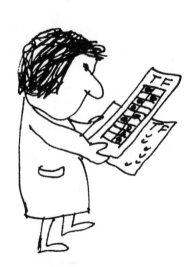

Computer scoring and analysis

In most major undergraduate and postgraduate examinations a computer is used to score and analyse objective-type examinations. You must therefore be familiar with the process and how to interpret the results. The students' marks may be

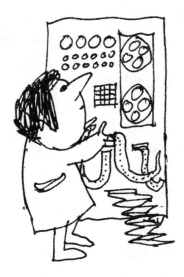

fed into the computer automatically from a marking machine or the raw marks may be fed in by card or via an interactive terminal. Most institutional computers have programs which will produce lists of student results in alphabetical order and in order of merit. Raw scores can be manipulated to produce, for example, percentage scores.

The computer will also generate statistical data about the examination. It can, for example, provide information on the number of questions answered by each student, the mean and standard deviation for the class and a reliability statistic such as a Kuder–Richardson test for internal consistency. If necessary the data can be re-worked to provide statistics on subsets of questions such as those covering separate topics.

The item analysis: This is a component of the computer print-out which warrants detailed discussion because of the problems it seems to cause many teachers. It contains valuable information for the person who has been responsible for constructing test times and assembling the examination. The item analysis provides numerical and statistical information on each item in the test.

A typical output of an item analysis for a multiple-choice question is shown in Figure 6.13.

FIGURE 6.13

EXAMPLE OF AN ITEM ANALYSIS

Percent correct of all students	Discrim- ination R biserial	Discrim- ination index	Difficulty index	Item no.
54.55	.39	.60	45.45	1
	Significant at 5.0% level Yes			

Number of students answering each alternative					
Group	Omitted	A	B	C*	D
Upper	1	0	0	39	2
Middle	4	0	0	31	35
Lower	6	3	5	14	14
TOTAL	11	3	5	84	51

*Correct answer

The **discrimination index** compares the performance of the students on the whole test with their performance on each item within the test. The students are divided on the basis of their performance on the test into upper, middle and lower groups. In most item analyses, for statistical reasons, the proportions happen to be 27%, 46% and 27% respectively. Looking at the example you will see that in the upper group 39 students answered correctly while in the lower group only 14 students answered correctly. The discrimination index is simply calculated from the following formula, which can almost as easily be done by hand as by computer.

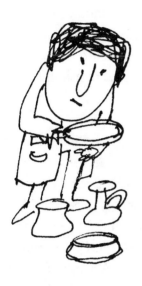

$$D = \frac{R_U - R_L}{\frac{1}{2}T}$$

Where R_U = number of students in upper group answering correctly

R_L = number of students in lower group answering correctly

T = total number of students answering correctly

$$\therefore D = \frac{39 - 14}{\frac{1}{2} \times 84} = \frac{25}{42} = 0.60$$

The discrimination index may have a value between +1 and -1. An item which did not discriminate between the two groups would produce an index of zero. An item where the lower group of students performed better than the top group of students would produce a negative index. Should the latter occur there is usually something seriously wrong with the item or there has been a technical or clerical error (e.g. the correct answer has been incorrectly indicated on the mark sheet or computer form). Generally speaking, one is looking for items to have a discrimination index of above 0.40, and certainly not less than 0.20, but an item should not necessarily be discarded because it fails to reach this level. It is always important to look at the content of the question when reviewing an item analysis.

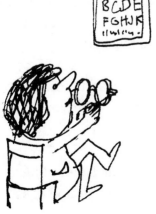

The discrimination R biserial (also known as the point-biserial correlation coefficient) provides information which is very similar to that provided by the discrimination index. A more sophisticated statistical approach correlates the relationship between the scores obtained on a particular item with the scores obtained on the test as a whole. A test of significance can be applied which is equivalent to a t-test of the difference between two means. High values indicate that students who performed well on the whole test also performed well on that item and that students who performed badly on the whole test also performed badly on that question. These values are meaningful only if they are significant at the 5% level. Interpretation of this statistic remains a matter for your judgement just as with the discrimination index.

The difficulty index is also calculated for you. It is simply the percentage of students who answered the item incorrectly. Some care is needed here as in some item analyses this term is used to express the percentage of students who answered correctly. In our example, such confusion should not arise as both are provided. An item difficulty index of around 30% or a percentage correct of around 70% is suggested for a one from five choice item with figures of 25% and 75% respectively for a one from four choice item.

The **efficiency of distractors** can be judged by inspecting the table. Only one of the distractors (D) attracted responses from the upper group, but all distractors (A, B & D) attracted responses from the lower group. However, distractor A only attracted three responses and has essentially converted a one from four MCQ into a one from three MCQ. The question should thus be reviewed and distractor A replaced with a more plausible alternative. Many questions will be found that are much worse than this where two or even three distractors serve no useful purpose.

5. DIRECT OBSERVATION

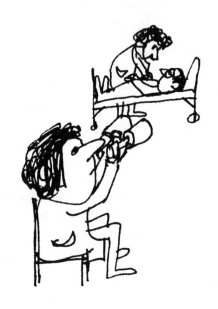

Direct observation of the student performing a technical or an interpersonal skill in the real, simulated or examination setting would appear to be the most valid way of assessing such skills. Unfortunately, the reliability of these observations is likely to be so low as to make such data almost worthless. This is particularly so in the complex interpersonal area where no alternative form of assessment is available. However, we must continue to make assessments of the student's history taking ability, doctor–patient relationship, counselling ability and so on, if only to indicate to the student our commitment to these vital skills. In doing so, you would be well advised to use the information predominantly for feedback purposes rather than for important decision making purposes.

Various ways have been suggested by which these limitations might be minimized. One is to improve the method of scoring and another is to improve the performance of the observer. The former involves the design of checklists and rating forms.

Checklists

A checklist is basically a two-point rating scale. The assessor has to decide whether each component on the list is present/absent; adequate/inadequate; satisfactory/unsatisfactory. Only if each component is very clearly defined and readily observable can a checklist be a reliable instrument. They are particularly useful for assessing technical skills. An example of such a form used to assess physical examination skills is shown in Figure 6.14. The key components which have made this particular checklist a reasonably reliable test are the clear instructions and the breakdown of the skill (the ability to assess vascular insufficiency in the lower limbs) into a series of subskills, each of which is observable.

FIGURE 6.14
EXAMPLE OF A
CLINICAL SKILLS
CHECKLIST

Examiner's instructions to students			
This patient presents with symptoms suggestive of intermittent claudication. Please examine the lower limbs from the cardiovascular point of view. Provide a commentary on what you are doing and what you have found.			
	Adequate	*Inadequate*	*Not performed*
1 Inspection (observes and comments on skin and colour changes)			
2 Palpation: a. Temperature b. Popliteal pulse c. Post. tibial pulse d. D. pedis pulse			
3 Circulation: a. Leg elevation b. Leg dependency			
4 Auscultation (femoral)			

Rating forms

Rating forms come in many styles. The essential feature is that the observer is required to make a judgement along a scale which may be continuous or intermittent. They are widely used to assess behaviour or performance because no other methods are available, but the subjectivity of the assessment is an unavoidable problem. Because of this, multiple independent rating of the same student on the same activity are essential if any sort of justice is to be done. The examples below show several alternative structures for rating the same ability. They are derived from published formats used to obtain information about ward performance of specialist trainees or interns. The component skill being assessed is 'Obtaining the data base' and only one subcomponent (obtaining information from the patient) is illustrated.

FIGURE 6·15
EXAMPLES OF RATING
FORMS

Format 1

	Top Quarter	Upper Middle Quarter	Lower Middle Quarter	Bottom Quarter
Obtaining information from the patient	4	3	2	1

Format 2

Obtaining information from the patient

☐	☐	☐	☐	☐
very effective	effective	reasonable	poor	inadequate

☐ unable to judge

Format 3

Obtaining information from the patient

Little or no information obtained	Some information obtained. Major errors or omissions	Adequate performance. Most information elicited.	Very thorough exploration of patient's problems.
☐	☐	☐	☐

Format 3 is the one we would recommend for two reasons. The first is that there is an attempt to provide descriptive anchor points which may be helpful in clarifying for the observer what standards should be applied. The second is a more pragmatic one. In a study we undertook, it was the format most frequently preferred by experienced clinical raters. Despite this preference we must say that the reliability achieved by our raters using this form, or any other form, was far from satisfactory. However, when you compare the broad nature of the skills being assessed in this type of rating form to the narrow and clearly defined skills being assessed in the checklist example then you will hardly be surprised at our results. Yet checklists of the type demonstrated in our example are rarely seen in use in medical schools and most rating forms are far less specific and less clearly defined than the examples given.

Improving the performance of the observer

It has often been claimed that training of raters will improve reliability. This seems to make sense but what evidence there is shows that training makes remarkably little difference. A recent study of our own suggested that a better approach might be to select raters who are inherently more consistent than others. Common sense dictates that observers should be adequately briefed on the rating form and that they should not be asked to rate on aspects of the student's performance that they have not observed. This may sound simple enough but studies have repeatedly shown that staff rarely observe students talking to patients, taking histories or performing full physical examinations, yet most seem happy enough to complete rating forms which required them to assess such skills.

6. ORAL

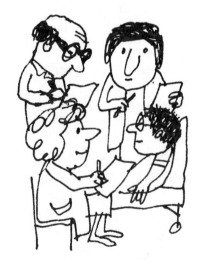

The oral or viva voce examination has for centuries been the predominant method, and sometimes the only method, used to assess medical students, particularly in the clinical area. The traditional oral, which gives considerable freedom to the examiner to vary the questions asked from student to student and to exercise personal bias, has consistently been shown in research studies to have severe deficiencies in terms of reliability. A major study, by the American National Board of Medical Examiners, of bedside oral examinations showed that correlation between examiners was overall no greater than would have occurred by chance.

Without doubt, face-to-face interaction between student and examiner provides a unique opportunity to test interactive skills which cannot be assessed in any other way. However, these skills are not usually the focus of attention and several studies have shown that the majority of questions in medical student oral examinations require little more than the recall of isolated fragments of information, something more easily and more reliably assessed by objective written tests.

We would recommend that reliance on oral examination be considerably reduced. Many of the activities currently assessed in oral examinations can be incorporated into the objective structured approach discussed in the next section. However, orals may be appropriate where one wishes to discriminate among top students where higher intellectual skills could be challenged by in-depth questioning.

Should you wish to retain oral examinations then certain steps should be undertaken to minimize the likely problems:

FIGURE 6.16
PROCEDURE FOR
CONDUCTING ORAL
EXAMINATIONS

Procedure

A Standardize the content:

- define the content to be tested

- if it is a theoretical oral get the examiners together beforehand and prepare a standard set of questions to be asked of each student. These should be identical if examined students can be kept apart from students yet to be examined. If not, the questions should be equivalent in content and difficulty

- if it is a clinical viva the same should apply but in this case the students should be faced with similar or equivalent patients and asked to perform the same task. There is no longer any place for allowing examiners the freedom of a room full of patients with a wide variety of conditions. The use of simulated patients has been used in some places to standardize the test situation.

B Reduce the examiner inconsistency:

- prepare structured marking sheets or rating forms and brief examiners in their use

- use as many examiners as possible. In other words, break down the oral examination into several shorter rather than one long session

- ask them to make sure each student gets asked the agreed questions and is given approximately the same time to answer them

- ensure that each examiner marks independently and avoids discussing individual students until all marks are correlated.

Surprising as it may seem, examiners used to traditional vivas seem to appreciate this structured approach as most are well aware of their own limitations. When the content is standardized they become much more confident of assessing the differences between students. Therefore, do not be frightened to suggest such changes, even in the most conservative medical school.

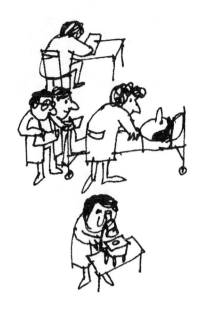

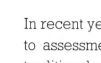
7. **STRUCTURED** (Clinical/Practical)

In recent years there has been a search for new approaches to assessment, particularly in the clinical area where the traditional methods have known deficiencies. One of the most interesting of these developments has been the structured clinical examination initially described by Harden and his colleagues in Dundee and subsequently developed by ourselves as an integral part of the final year examinations. The structured examination is not really an assessment method but rather an administrative structure in which a variety of test methods can be incorporated. The aim is to test a wide range of skills in an objective fashion.

The students rotate through a series of stations and undertake a variety of tasks. An example of the stations used in one of our final year examinations is shown in Figure 6.17.

Marking sheets for the short-answer questions and checklists are prepared beforehand to improve the reliability of the scoring. All students are thus examined on the same content and marked on the same criteria by the same examiners. These are the features which are so different to those of traditional clinical examinations and vivas.

Though such examinations are particularly well suited to the clinical area, the method can be applied to any area where practical skills have to be assessed. As in any form of assessment, the definition of the content to be tested and the preparation of good test items is essential if a high degree of validity and reliability are to be obtained.

Should you wish to consider introducing such an approach you should read the articles given in the references.

8. **SELF-ASSESSMENT**

By 'self-assessment' we are not referring only to self-marking or to the use of multiple-choice questions to determine one's medical knowledge. We are referring to an assessment system which involves the students in establishing the criteria and standards they will apply to their work and then have them make judgments about the degree to which they have been met.

FIGURE 6.17

OUTLINE OF A STRUCTURED
CLINICAL EXAMINATION

Station	Task	Type of assessment			Time (min)
1	Examination of a urinary sediment	Short answer question			5
2	Interpretation of an ECG	"	"	"	5
3	Interpretation of a chest X-ray	"	"	"	5
4	Writing a prescription	"	"	"	5
5	Writing nursing orders	"	"	"	5
6	Fundal examination	"	"	"	5
7	Interpretation of heart sounds	"	"	"	5
8	Advice to diabetic on change in insulin regime	"	"	"	5
9	Interpretation of biochemical analysis	"	"	"	5
10	Interpretation of blood picture	"	"	"	5
11	Selection of oxygen masks	"	"	"	5
12	Post operative fluid orders	"	"	"	5
13	Cardiovascular assessment of the hypertensive patient	Direct observation using a checklist			10
14	Case write-up of station 13	Checklist			10
15	Examination of the breast	Direct observation using a checklist			10
				TOTAL	90

The skill of being able to make realistic evaluations of the quality of one's work is a skill that every graduating doctor should have. Yet, in conventional medical schools, few provide systematic opportunities for self-assessment skills to be learnt and developed. However, this form of evaluation is usually a fundamental component of the educational approach used by the new problem-based medical schools discussed in Chapter 5.

The introduction of self-assessment practices into existing courses has been shown to be feasible and desirable. Whether marks generated in this way should count towards a final grade is an undecided issue. Nevertheless, there is little doubt that self-assessment used primarily to help the students' understanding of their own ability and performance is worthwhile educationally and encourages openness and honesty about assessment.

If you wish to embark on a trial scheme you must first set about the task of establishing criteria and standards. This can be done at a series of small group meetings attended by staff and students. Both must agree on the criteria to be applied to the students' work. To help focus on this task you might have students reflect on questions such as:

★ How would you distinguish good from inadequate work?

★ What would characterize a good assignment in this course?

Once criteria have been specified, students use them to judge their own performance. Marks are awarded with reference to each criterion and a statement justifying the mark should be included. An alternative is to contrast their own mark with one given to them by a peer. The teacher may also mark a random sample to establish controls and to discourage cheating or self-delusion.

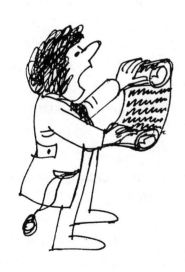

REPORTING THE RESULTS OF ASSESSMENT

In many major examinations you will be required to report the results as a final mark or grade based on a number of different assessment methods. What usually happens is that marks from these different assessments are simply added or averaged and the final mark or grade awarded. Simple though this approach may be, it can introduce serious distortions. Factors contributing to this problem may be differing distributions of marks in each subtest; varying numbers of questions; differing levels of difficulty; and a failure to appropriately weight each component.

The answer is to convert each raw subscore to a standardized score. This is not the place to do more than alert you to the need to do so and refer you to a text on educational measurement (e.g. Mehrens and Lehmann) or to advise you to enlist the aid of an educational statistician, who can usually be found by contacting the teaching unit in your institution.

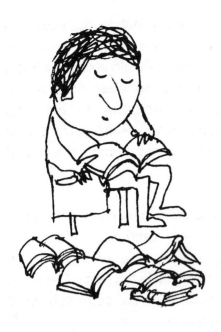

GUIDED READING

There are many useful general texts on educational measurement. Two which provide a straightforward account of the principles and procedures of assessment are W.A. Mehrens and I.J. Lehmann's *Measurement and Evaluation in Education and Psychology* (third edition), Holt, Rinehart and Winston, New York, 1984 and R.L. Ebel's *Essentials of Educational Measurement* (third edition), Prentice Hall, Englewood Cliffs, New Jersey, 1979. Both have useful discussions of broad assessment considerations such as objectives, planning, realiability, validity and scoring, and also provide a wide range of examples of test items. J.P. Hubbard's book *Measuring Medical Education*, Lea and Febiger, Philadelphia, 1971, is also a useful resource.

We also list below references to some of the more recent methods of assessment, particularly those that are of specific interest in medical education.

Handbook of Written Simulations: their Construction and Analysis by C. H. McGuire, L. M. Solomon and P. G. Bashook, Centre for Educational Development, University of Illinois, Chicago, 1972. This is one of the few comprehensive accounts of the method of constructing a PMP of the branching type.

There are many variations of this technique but details of their preparation are hard to come by. There are many articles in the recent literature dealing with the issue of the validity and scoring of PMPs. One of our own articles could be used as an entry point (*Patient Management Problems: Issues of Validity*, D.I. Newble, J. Hoare and A. Baxter, Medical Education, 16, 1982: 137–142).

Problem Centred Learning: the Modified Essay Question in Medical Education by K. Hodgkin and J.D.E. Knox, Churchill-Livingstone, Edinburgh, 1975.
This is the book written by the originators of this method of assessment. It gives details and examples of how such questions should be constructed. An abbreviated version is available in the form of a booklet (No. 5) from the Association for the Study of Medical Education (ASME).

Assessment of Medical Competence Using a Structured Clinical Examination by R. M. Harden and F. A. Gleeson. This is available as an ASME booklet (No. 8) and can also be found in journal form in Medical Education, 13, 1979: 44–54. It provides details of how to construct such an examination and contains plenty of examples.

A New Approach to the Final Examination in Medicine and Surgery by D. I. Newble and R. G. Elmslie, Lancet, 2, 1981: 517–518. This article provides a brief account of our own work using the structured type of examination to assess the clinical competence of medical students.

Assessing Clinical Competence by V.R. Neufeld and G.R. Norman, Springer, New York, 1985, is a multiauthor state-of-the art review. It looks in depth at all the methods being used in the evaluation of competence as well as dealing with broader issues.

7: PREPARING TEACHING MATERIALS AND USING TEACHING AIDS

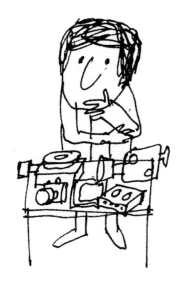

INTRODUCTION

In your teaching career you will use quite a wide range of audio visual and printed teaching materials. How these materials can be economically and effectively produced and how you might use them is the focus of this chapter.

Perhaps the most fundamental criterion for judging the effectiveness of your teaching material is its audibility and/or visibility. If that seems too obvious to warrant mention, have a look at some of the materials used by others: sound recordings that are so distorted that they cannot be understood, slides with excessive amounts of tiny detail that cannot be read on the screen, blackboards that look like someone's doodle pad, and faded handouts that cannot be read. Exaggeration? It does happen! When it does, it seriously interferes with the effectiveness of teaching. Attention to the way in which the material is produced and how it is used in teaching will eliminate many of these problems.

BASIC PRINCIPLES OF TEACHING MATERIAL PREPARATION

Whether you are preparing a simple handout or a video-cassette, there are some basic principles that can be incorporated into your design and preparation that will enhance the quality and effectiveness of the material.

Relevance

Materials should be relevant to the purpose for which they were created and to the students' level of understanding of the topic. Complex handouts distributed at the end of a lecture and never referred to by the teacher are a classic offender of this principle.

Linkage

An introduction is usually required to establish the purpose of the material and to link it with what it is reasonable to expect students to already know.

Simplicity

Simplicity in the use of language and design, the avoidance of needless qualifications and the use of suitable abstractions of complex situations can be positive aids to understanding. For example, a simple line diagram of the structure of the heart may be more helpful in an explanation than a full colour photograph.

Emphasis

Emphatic 'signs' can be incorporated into all teaching materials to stress important ideas, to indicate a change in the development of an argument, or to identify new material. Examples of emphasis include headings and underlinings in print, the use of colour on charts and slides, the use of pointers and close-ups in video, and statements such as 'this is a major factor' on a sound recording.

Consistency in the use of pattern and style

Students acquire a 'feel' for the particular style you use to present material. Needless changing of style is only going to confuse them. This is one of the reasons why imported materials, such as video recordings, often achieve less impact than similar materials produced by a local teacher.

TYPES OF TEACHING MATERIAL AND AIDS

With these basic principles in mind, the preparation and use of several basic types of teaching materials and aids will now be described. These are:

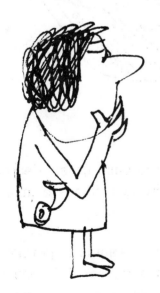

1	The overhead projector
2	The blackboard and whiteboard
3	The 35 mm slide projector
4	Video and film
5	Tape-slide presentations
6	Printed materials

This list is by no means exhaustive. In keeping with the general thrust of this book, the intention is mainly to get you started and to help you develop some confidence in this aspect of your teaching work.

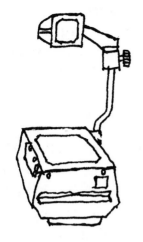

1. **THE OVERHEAD PROJECTOR**

This valuable visual aid can project a wide range of transparency materials and silhouettes of opaque objects onto a screen positioned behind the teacher. Because it can project both written and diagrammatic information, it reduces your need to engage in detailed descriptions and increases the opportunities for discussion with students. It also allows you to indicate things on the transparency without turning your back to the audience, an advantage over using a slide projector.

The full benefit of the overhead projector will not be realized in your teaching unless you give careful attention to three things: the preparation of the transparency, the way the projector is set up in a room or lecture theatre, and the way you actually use it. We shall now turn to a consideration of each of these matters.

Transparency preparation

Figure 7.1 shows what a transparency looks like. It consists of an acetate sheet mounted onto a cardboard frame. Additional sheets of acetate on the same frame are known as overlays.

FIGURE 7·1
EXAMPLE OF
TRANSPARENCY

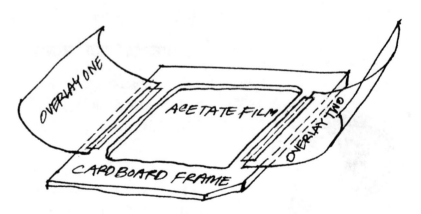

Overlays are particularly helpful to build up an idea as a presentation develops. The following methods of making transparencies are available:

Felt pens: felt pens containing water soluble or permanent ink are available for making transparencies. Information is printed or drawn directly onto an acetate sheet. A suggested procedure is to mount the acetate sheet onto a frame with adhesive tape, place a piece of ruled paper underneath the acetate as a guide and write onto the sheet. Another sheet of

5MM LETTERS

clean paper placed under your hand will prevent smudges appearing on the acetate. Printing should be no smaller than 5 mm in height and preferably larger. Use black, blue, brown or green pens for lettering, avoiding red, orange and yellow which are difficult to read at a distance.

Adhesive films and letters: you can use rub-down materials such as Letraset directly onto an acetate sheet if you wish to give a professional looking finish. This is time consuming if you have to do it yourself and should be restricted to the preparation of transparencies to be used repeatedly or in prestigious meetings. A much easier method is to use a lettering machine. With this device, bold letters are punched out onto a clear tape and then transferred to the transparency. Materials prepared in these ways are best used in conjunction with one of the following processes.

Thermal copying: thermal copiers offer an economical means of producing transparencies providing your original is of good quality, with bold black lettering and thick black lines. There are a variety of thermal films from which to select. These will provide black images on a clear or coloured background. Two or more colours can be combined in one transparency with interesting effects. Information on specific films and the procedure you should follow is supplied by manufacturers or can be obtained from a visual aid consultant.

Photocopying: many plain paper copiers will now accept acetate sheets, enabling the production of black and white transparencies at the touch of a button. It is essential that the type of sheet selected is suitable for use with the copier available and that the original material is large and clear. Lettering, for example, must be at least 5 mm in height. Avoid the temptation to make overheads directly from books or from ordinary typed materials. If you wish to use such material you should make an enlargement. This is now possible on several photocopying machines. An alternative is to photograph the original, get it enlarged and use this to produce the transparency.

Graphics and word-processing packages: micro-computer software packages give you a means of producing master sheets for transparencies. Graphics packages allow you to prepare diagrams as well. Provided the printout is of sufficient quality (a laser printer is best) and large fonts are chosen in setting-up the page, excellent transparencies can be produced.

Other uses of the overhead projector: there are other, less orthodox ways in which you can use the overhead projector. Silhouettes of cardboard cut-outs or solid objects can be projected onto the screen. These may be co-ordinated with a prepared transparency. Transparent or translucent materials such as liquids in test tubes or biological specimens mounted on, or contained in, clear containers can be prepared.

The following are points which should be kept in mind when preparing an overhead transparency.

FIGURE 7.2
GUIDELINES FOR MAKING
AN EFFECTIVE OVER-
HEAD TRANSPARENCY

> **Guidelines**
>
> ★ Limit each transparency to one main idea. Several simple transparencies are preferable to a complicated one.
>
> ★ Reduce tabulated data to essential or to rounded figures. A single graph or diagram may be preferable.
>
> ★ Typed originals must be photographed and enlarged. To help in this, use a typing template – a bold rectangular outline with an aspect ratio of 4:3. An outline measuring 120 mm wide and 90 mm high is suitable for this.
>
> ★ As an alternative, or as a supplement to typing, consider using a lettering machine or Letraset.

Setting up and using the overhead projector

In some situations you will have flexibility in setting up the projector and screen. It is usual to place the projector so that it is adjacent to the lectern or table from which you are working. Ensure that the projected image is square on the screen and free from angular and colour distortions. Angular distortions in the vertical axis can be overcome by tilting the top of the screen forward. Colour distortions, such as red or blue in the corners of the projected image, can usually be remedied by making an adjustment to the lamp. A control for this is often inside the projector. It is important to turn the electricity off at the power point before the adjustment is attempted.

Whenever a projector is moved, or before a presentation is commenced, the focus and position of the image must be checked. Once this is done, it is usually unnecessary to look at the screen again, particularly if you use a pen or pointer

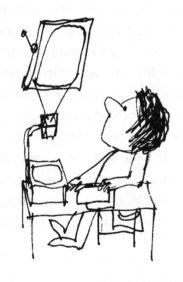

directly on the transparency. This enables you to maintain eye-contact with students. If you wish to mask out part of the transparency, place a sheet of paper between the film and the glass stage of the projector; the weight of the transparency should prevent the paper from moving or falling away.

Remember to allow students plenty of time to read what you have projected. Many teachers find this difficult to do. One way is to carefully read the transparency to yourself word for word. As well, make sure anything you have to say complements the transparency. Do not expect students to listen to you and to look at something on the screen that is only vaguely related to what is being said. It is advisable to have the lamp on only when a transparency is being used in your teaching, otherwise the projected image or the large area of white light will distract the students' attention.

Storage of transparencies

Your transparencies will last many years if carefully used and stored, so the effort in making them carefully and professionally is well worthwhile. A dust and scratch free environment is best for storage. You can use the cardboard boxes that the mounts are sold in for this or make a protective wallet from two manilla folders sealed together with tape. Large X-ray film boxes are also ideal for storage. Some teachers store a whole lecture in this way and interleave their transparencies with their lecture notes.

2. THE BLACKBOARD

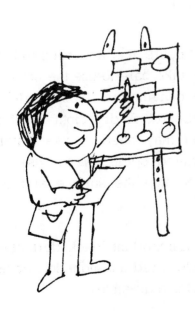

The blackboard (which these days may be green) is still a commonly used visual aid and the one that you are likely to use quite frequently, unless you rely exclusively on the overhead projector. Few teachers give much thought to the material they put on the board or to the way they use it. This is a pity. The results of the work are often ugly and indecipherable. Well planned and well used blackboard work is a delight to see and is a valuable ally in conveying information accurately and clearly to your students.

Preparation

It is important to think ahead about your use of the board and make suitable notations in your teaching notes. Plan your use of the board by dividing the available space into a number of sections. Each section is then used for a specific purpose such as references, diagrams, a summary of the structure of the lecture and so on.

Using a blackboard

The following are some guidelines for using a blackboard.

FIGURE 7·3
GUIDELINES FOR USING A BLACKBOARD

Guidelines

- Start a presentation with a clean board. Downward strokes with a duster will prevent wide spreading of chalk dust.

- Try to avoid talking and writing on the blackboard at the same time. When speaking, look at students, not at the board.

- Face the board squarely and move across the board when writing. This will assist in writing horizontally.

- Stand aside when writing or drawing is completed to enable students to see the blackboard.

- Concise information in skeleton note form is preferred to a 'newspaper' effect.

- Underline headings and important or unfamiliar words to give visual emphasis.

- Always give students a chance to copy down the information you have taken time to put on the blackboard (if it is intended that they should have a copy).

- Use colours liberally but with discretion. Yellow and white are suitable colours for most written work. Use red, dark blue and green chalk sparingly as they are difficult to see and difficult to erase.

The whiteboard

The same principles of blackboard use and preparation apply also to whiteboards. Do take care to use the correct pens with a whiteboard as some can ruin its surface. Also take care when cleaning a whiteboard. A dry cloth is often adequate but sometimes you may need to use water, detergent or perhaps methylated spirits. Never use an abrasive cleaner as it will scratch the surface and do irreparable damage.

The colour of the pens you use is important. Black, dark blue and green are best. Avoid yellow, red and light colours as these can be difficult to read from a distance.

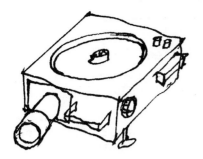

3. **THE 35 mm SLIDE PROJECTOR**

Much of what has been said about the overhead projector applies to slide projection. However, you will recognize that there are important differences between the two and that one of these is that full colour images can be used in slides. This may be an advantage but with some students it may also be a disadvantage unless their level of understanding is sufficient to enable them to see what is relevant and pertinent in the material you are using. Slide interpretation can be aided by including in the photograph an appropriate reference point or a scale. Remember that a slide that is suitable for a meeting of medical specialists may be quite inappropriate for a group of students.

Slide preparation

The major error in slide making is to assume that legibility in one medium, such as a table in a book or a journal, ensures slide legibility. Slides made from printed materials frequently contain too much detail and fine line work to enable them to be projected satisfactorily. This means that you may have to have artwork redrawn and new lettering added. Check any slides in your possession for legibility. A useful rule of thumb is that a slide which can be read without a magnifier is generally satisfactory. A better method is to go with a colleague to a large lecture theatre, project your slides and check to see if all details are legible and understandable.

When making slides avoid the temptation to put all the details into the slide. If it is important for students to have all the details, provide them in a handout so that they can refer to it and keep it for reference. This ensures that they have accurate information on hand.

University or hospital photographers will advise you on the different processes available to produce your slides. These processes will usually include simple black-on-white slides, colour slides and diazo slides (white against blue, green or red backgrounds, the blue being preferred for clarity). Another attractive way to prepare slides is to obtain negatives (white on black) and colour the white sections in by hand using coloured marking pens. The possibility exists for using separate colours to highlight different points on the slide. Whatever you choose, try to achieve a degree of consistency by sticking to one type of slide. Guidelines for the preparation of effective slides are given below.

FIGURE 7·4
GUIDELINES FOR
MAKING EFFECTIVE
SLIDES

Guidelines

➡ Limit each slide to one main idea.

➡ Reduce tabulated data to essential or to rounded figures. Simple graphs and diagrams are to be preferred.

➡ When making new slides use a template with an aspect ratio of 3:2. An outline for typing of about 140 mm × 95 mm or 230 mm × 150 mm for artwork is suitable.

Setting up and using the slide projector

Slide projection equipment is normally part of the standard fixtures in a lecture theatre these days so the question of setting up does not usually arise. If it does, however, locate the projector and screen with care to give the best view to students and so that it is convenient for you to operate the projector and room lights with a minimum of fuss. A remote control device will be an invaluable aid.

Slide projection

Before loading your slides into a cartridge or carousel, carefully plan the sequence of their use. If your teaching is to be interspersed with slides, consider using black slides to separate your material and to avoid having to keep turning the projector on and off or leaving an inappropriate slide on view. Black slides are simply pieces of opaque film mounted in a slide frame to block off light to the screen and can be easily made from exposed X-ray film. If you plan to use the same slide on more than one occasion during a presentation, arrange to have duplicates made to save you and your students the agony of having to search back and forth through a slide series.

It is essential to have your slides marked or 'spotted' for projection (see Figure 7.5).

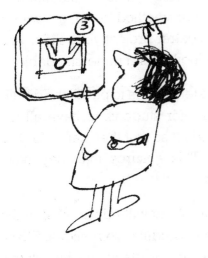

FIGURE 7·5

PROCEDURE FOR "SPOTTING" SLIDES

Procedure

1 Place your slides on a light box (an overhead projector is ideal for this) so that the image is the same way up as it is to appear on the screen.

2 Turn slide upside down.

3 Mark or number the slide in the top righthand corner.

As a check, the slides should be upside down and emulsion side (i.e. the dull side) towards the screen.

When showing your slides, it is rarely necessary to turn off all the lights. Remember that students may wish to take notes and so you should plan to leave some light on or to dim the main lights. Further helpful advice on using slides is given in the chapter on presenting a paper at a scientific meeting.

4. VIDEO AND FILM

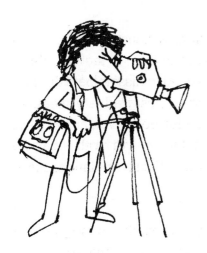

Of all the teaching materials at your disposal you will probably find that video and, to a less extent, film, will give you the most flexibility and the opportunity to experiment with novel approaches to teaching. This is particularly true of the material you make yourself but you should become familiar with the range of suitable commercially available materials before embarking on a career as a producer. You will find that the medical area has been particularly well catered for in this regard. Pharmaceutical companies often have very useful videos and film available for use in medical education.

Although the uses of video and film are similar, video does offer you several additional advantages such as ease of production and relative cheapness. These have tended to make this medium rather more popular and flexible than film. Incidentally, it is important to explain what we mean by 'video' and to distinguish video from 'television'. Television generally refers to the process of transmitting and receiving pictures and sound via broadcast. Television programmes are made in large studios with elaborate production systems or they may be broadcast films. Television has had some educational uses but because of rigid time scheduling of broadcasts and the cost it has not found much acceptance. This has changed to some extent with the arrival of the video cassette recorder which has enabled broadcasts to be recorded for later use but this, of course, is usually in breach of copyright laws. Video is a term applied to locally made material produced in a university or hospital studio or by the teacher using a single camera and recorder system. It is usually of a lesser technical standard than broadcast television. Video is generally produced with a restricted audience in mind.

Using video and film in teaching

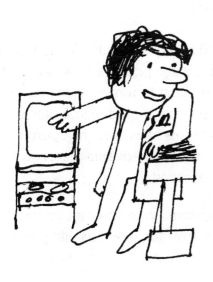

As with many teaching aids the uses are restricted only by your imagination and by the resources at your disposal. Some of the potential uses of video and film are described below.

As introductory material: video and film can be used at the start of a course or series of lectures to stimulate interest, to provide an overview and to form a basis for further teaching. For example, a film on the effects of cigarette smoking could be used as a point of departure for a discourse on lung cancer.

As a major source of information: a constant flow of new drugs, techniques and procedures are a fact of life in medicine. Video and film can be used to disseminate this new information to your students and to postgraduate meetings with which you may be involved. A further advantage of these media is that they can provide the viewer with vicarious experience where this might be difficult or dangerous to obtain at first hand.

As a means of modelling: this use is similar to the previous one, but you may find it helpful to produce material which demonstrates a technique or procedure in a clear step-by-step manner that students can watch and emulate at their own pace. An example might be a demonstration of how a physical examination should be done.

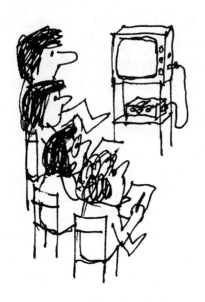

As a stimulus for discussion: short open-ended sections of video or film can be made to stimulate discussion among students (trigger films). For example, in the space of a minute or two, a video can show a patient asking questions or making personal remarks about the doctor. Students respond to the material as it is presented and the stimulus and the response is then discussed. This we have found to be valuable for starting discussion about attitudes dealing with emotional situations. Sometimes it is possible to locate suitable stimulus material in old films that would otherwise have no use. Trigger films are commercially available.

As a means of distribution and relay: carefully placed video cameras can be used to distribute pictures to a separate viewing room or even to relay them to remote locations. An obvious example of this is their use in operating theatres to enable a larger number of students to witness the operation. Such an approach certainly provides advantages over the lecture theatre galleries of yesteryear.

As an information storage system: video has an important role to play in storing information for later teaching or for research use. For example, a recording can be made (with permission) of a particularly interesting clinical case or of a doctor–patient interview for subsequent review and analysis. This approach we use extensively for training students in history taking as we described in the chapter on course design.

As a means of assembling visual and audio information: video can be extremely helpful if you want to assemble a variety of information in one 'package'. Film clips, stills, models, interviews, recorded sounds and graphics can be recorded, assembled and edited to make a teaching programme. You will need to obtain the advice of your audio-visual department before embarking on such a project.

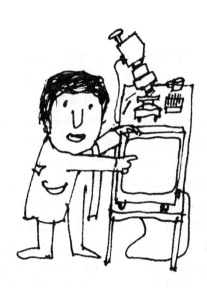

As a magnification medium: many medical teachers find that video is a handy tool to 'blow-up' the action or to display pictures of pathological specimens. These can, of course, be recorded if needed for subsequent use.

These examples of video and film use are by no means exhaustive nor are they mutually exclusive in their application. For example, in teaching oral pathology, video is used to magnify materials, to distribute and display it in a large laboratory (thus ensuring that all students are seeing the same thing) and sometimes to record the information as a source for student self-study.

The advent of the home video and the video disc are an indication that video, like the computer, is destined to play a larger role in education. Our experience with producing video discs is that this medium provides two significant advantages for the medical teacher. First, because of its enormous visual storage capacity, the disc can be used to bank large numbers of clinical slides, X-rays and film or video sequences in a readily accessible and durable way. Second, when used with a computer, the student can work interactively with the visual material. The exploration of this exciting development is just beginning for medical education. Video discs for this purpose are expensive to produce but copies are relatively cheap. They are now becoming available commercially.

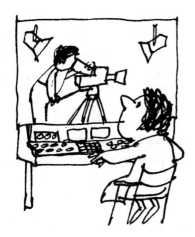

Making educational videos

In this section it is assumed that you have been asked or have decided to make a video to illustrate some aspect of your teaching. Depending on the complexity of the proposal, you may use a simple camera and recorder system available in your department or decide to use the services of an audio-visual unit. In the latter case you will be able to draw on their guidance in going about the production. Nevertheless, there are a number of considerations in making a video which are outlined here to prepare you for discussions with producers from the unit or, alternatively, to help you undertake the work on your own.

Planning: as with most educational situations, careful planning will repay dividends in production time and in the quality of the product. The first step in planning is to commit your thoughts to paper by writing down the story line. This is simply a statement of the main message you wish to communicate in your programme. The story line can be as brief as a sentence or two but should be no more than half a page or so in length. You may wish to sketch in some ideas to help you visualize the content. Once you are satisfied with your story line, turn your attention to reviewing the educational, technical and administrative considerations in producing and using the video in your teaching. We have found it helpful to pose a series of questions to focus on these considerations.

The **educational** questions are these:
* what are students expected to learn by viewing the proposed video?
* how is the topic taught at present?
* why is video being substituted for the present method of teaching?
* is video an appropriate medium to achieve the aims?
* how will the proposed video be used in teaching? (e.g. will students be expected to carry out any discussion or exercises after viewing it?)
* will the material be suitable for the students' level of understanding and skill?
* how will the effectiveness of the video be assessed?

The **technical** questions are:
➡ is the technical quality of the production and playback equipment adequate to show the detail and colour you require?

➡ in what format is the finished video required? (U-Matic, VHS, Beta, or video disc will be the main alternatives here).

➡ are the technical resources available to you adequate for the task?

➡ are additional material such as graphics, slides and sound effects required?

Finally, the important **administrative** questions to consider are:

● are there sufficient resources of people, equipment and money available to undertake the work?

● when is the finished work required?

● who (if not yourself) is to accept responsibility for the production?

● is the production timetable clear to all parties involved and realistic in terms of other commitments?

These, then, are some of the questions you need to consider before embarking on your work. If you intend to work alone, it will be helpful to discuss at least the educational questions with a colleague and you may need to seek some advice on a number of technical matters.

Scripting: the script is the detailed plan of your programme. It indicates the relationship between visuals and commentary. The script is used to guide those making the programme in such things as visual sequences, narration, materials required and so on.

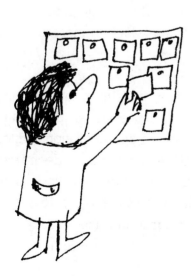

In preparing a script, you will find the use of blank white cards invaluable. Visual ideas and notes for the commentary can be sketched onto the cards. The cards can then be arranged into the best sequence. Try, as much as you can, to think visually. Use sketches rather than written notes to help you. Remember, you are employing a visual medium so let it work to best advantage for you. If you find that there seems to be a large amount of talk in your developing script, critically review what you have done and perhaps consider using a sound cassette instead.

Incidentally, what is meant by the 'best sequence'? There are several ways in which you might go about answering this question, always, of course, with your content and students in mind. Desirable ways of sequencing ideas are to proceed from what students already know to what they don't know, from simple ideas to complex ones, from a whole view to a part view and from concrete ideas to abstract ideas.

The sequenced cards can then be used as the basis to write your script. The exact format of your script will depend on the complexity of the production resources at your disposal.

Recording: before you commence recording, you must check that all participants in your project know what is expected of them, that all equipment is working satisfactorily and that the subject is well lit. A rehearsal will help you here. Video playback allows you to check your work as you go, a distinct advantage over film.

As you work try to keep the following points in mind:

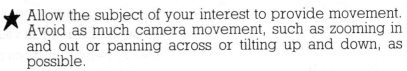
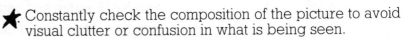

> **Guidelines**
>
> ★ Allow the subject of your interest to provide movement. Avoid as much camera movement, such as zooming in and out or panning across or tilting up and down, as possible.
>
> ★ Constantly check the composition of the picture to avoid visual clutter or confusion in what is being seen.
>
> ★ Remember that you are also recording sound and that this should be as clear as possible at all times.

Editing: your recordings will usually need to be edited by using electronic video editing equipment. Editing is simply a process of selecting and joining together visual sequences in the order dictated by your script. When editing is complete, you will need to add a sound track which is most likely to include your narration.

Reviewing your programme: once the euphoria of having completed your first recording has passed, sit down and critically review your work and make any alterations which are technically necessary and educationally desirable. When you first use the recording with students collect some information from them as well. A useful ploy is to watch students as they go through the programme. You will often be able to pick up sections that are causing difficulty or confusion.

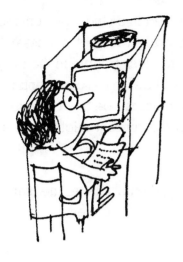

5. TAPE-SLIDE PRESENTATIONS

Tape-slide programmes are an effective way of presenting material to medical students. They are also cheaper than video programmes and much simpler to prepare. Unless movement is essential to your message then always consider a tape-slide presentation before a video presentation. It is usual to devise the programme in such a way that students can work alone and at their own pace.

Visual information in the programme is presented on 35 mm slides and a commentary on a sound cassette guides and explains. In some tape-slide equipment, electronic pulses can be put on the cassette tape which will change slides automatically.

Before embarking on the production be sure to consult the section in this chapter on slide preparation. Most of the principles for making an educational videocassette apply to making tape-slide programmes and you are directed back to that material for details. Briefly the main principles are:

Planning: this includes writing a story line, considering educational, technical and administrative questions and preparing a script.

Scripting: the commentary you prepare should be in simple spoken English. Avoid reading from an over-formal text and avoid indirect references such as 'these', 'they' and 'it', which may create confusion. We have found it best to use a conversational mode imagining that you are talking to a single person. All too often tape-slide programmes are like recorded lectures. Your commentary can be made more interesting by the planned use of questions, pauses for student thinking, pre-recorded sound effects or interviews, and deliberate breaks in which short exercises or problems can be tackled. Make sure the visual content on the screen matches the commentary. A mismatch between the visual input and the audio input will inevitably cause confusion. Part of the script from a series of tape-slide programmes on electrocardiography is shown in Figure 7.7.

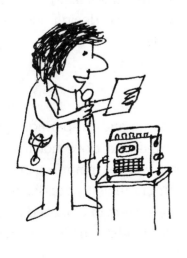

Recording: this requires much less in the way of technical expertise and facilities than video recording. A quiet room and a good quality tape recorder are all that is required, though better quality can be obtained in a studio. Automatic slide changing impulses can be added later if necessary. However, it is just as easy, and often less trouble in the long run, to include a request to change slides in the commentary. This then ensures that the programme can be used with less sophisticated equipment such as the student might have at home.

Reviewing the programme: you should make the same critical review of the presentation as suggested in the preceding section on video.

FIGURE 7.7
PART OF A SCRIPT
FROM A TAPE-SLIDE
PROGRAMME

VISUAL	AUDIO
SLIDE 1. TITLE	THIS IS THE THIRD OF A SERIES OF TUTORIALS ON ELECTROCARDIOGRAPHY. YOU SHOULD NOW HAVE THE TITLE SLIDE SHOWING AND CORRECTLY FOCUSSED (PAUSE). LET US REVIEW SOME OF THE IMPORTANT POINTS YOU HAVE LEARNED FROM THE FIRST TWO SESSIONS.
SLIDE 2. ECG COMPLEXES	FIRST OF ALL, HOW'S YOUR TERMINOLOGY? HERE YOU SEE A LEFT-SIDED LEAD AND A RIGHT SIDED LEAD. JUST STOP THE TAPE FOR A MINUTE OR TWO AND WRITE DOWN WHAT THESE SYMBOLS MEAN THEN RESTART THE TAPE TO CONTINUE.
SLIDE 3.	HERE IS WHAT YOU SHOULD HAVE WRITTEN. "P" REPRESENTS ATRIAL DEPOLARIZATION ...

6. PRINTED MATERIALS

Books, journals, handouts and study guides carry a very large part of the instructional burden in teaching. Yet, often, surprisingly little thought is given to the design and use of these important teaching materials.

Design

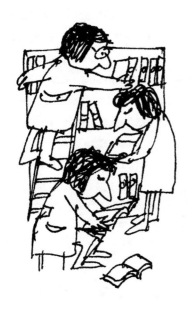

Care needs to be taken in designing and preparing printed materials. Over-organization of the text does not help the reader and may actually interfere with learning. You may find it helpful to yourself and to your students to standardize on layouts and perhaps to institute a system of coloured papers for different kinds of material (e.g. white for lecture notes, green for bibliographies, yellow for exercises). The basic principle for layout and design of printed materials are outlined below.

FIGURE 7.8
GUIDELINES FOR THE LAYOUT AND DESIGN OF PRINTED MATERIAL

Guidelines

Learning from printed materials can be enhanced by incorporating:

- an introduction to relate the new material to the past experience of the student
- a summary of the major ideas or arguments presented
- the use of major and minor headings
- space between paragraphs and sections to relieve the impact of too much print
- space for students to make annotations or notes
- simplicity in expression
- appropriately labelled illustrations, tables and graphs (a series of diagrams building up to a complete concept may be more helpful than one detailed diagram)
- questions and exercises within the text to stimulate thinking

---

Care also needs to be taken in choosing a suitable typeface. For example, text printed in sanserif typeface is somewhat more difficult to read than the standard serif print.

The variety of typefaces available for electric typewriters also make it necessary to select with care. Have a look at typographical layouts in better quality newspapers and journals for ideas that you can put into practice.

Using printed material

Handouts can serve a number of useful purposes in your teaching, but this medium is frequently mis-used because the material is often simply distributed to students and then quickly forgotten.

Handouts can be used by students as a note-taking guide to a lecture. Supplementary information, or perhaps a copy of a paper you think is important, can also be given in a handout. How you use the handout in your teaching is a crucial matter. We recommend that your students' attention be directed to the handout through the use of ploys such as discussing a particular definition, reading through a brief list of points with students, or getting them to fill in some part of it with additional information. If your students have to use the handout in the teaching session, it is likely they will remember it and not simply file it away to be forgotten.

Prescribed reading

Prescribed reading of textbooks and medical journals is another matter that warrants your careful attention. Some teachers swamp their students with lists of books and articles to be read with little thought about how they might manage the task. If you want the students to undertake some reading, then consider the following points:

★ what are students expected to achieve by undertaking the reading?
(make this purpose clearly known to the students)
★ how will the reading be followed up in subsequent teaching?
★ will the recommended reading be readily available in libraries or through bookshops?
★ how can the reading be usefully organized?
(arrange the material in a logical fashion, indicate why an item has been listed and what is especially important about it)

NEW TECHNOLOGIES

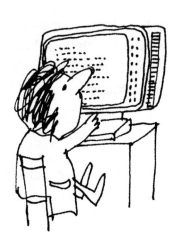

The microelectronics revolution has yet to make a major impact on medical education but it must inevitably do so in the near future. How it will do so is hard to predict and it is not within the scope of this book to consider the matter in detail. The growing number of households with sophisticated video equipment and computers will dramatically change the availability of information and educational materials at present restricted by limited access to libraries and audio-visual resource centres.

Anything written about computers and microcomputers will inevitably be out of date by the time it is published. However, in the educational arena it is not the technology that will be a critical factor but our ability to use and adapt it to our defined educational purposes. Computers have been used quite widely in medical education for some years particularly for computer-aided instruction, computer-based simulation, problem solving exercises of varying complexities and computerized self-assessment programmes. Despite many pilot projects, such applications are not widely available, often being dependent on the presence or absence of an enthusiastic staff member. If you are such an enthusiast you probably know more about the subject than we do. If you are not, but see potential for the use of a computer in your teaching, then you should seek the advice of your own computing centre.

Perhaps one of the more predictable uses of the ubiquitous silicon chip is in the area of information storage. It has been estimated that an average book can be reduced to about two million 'bits' of information, a storage capacity well within the capacity of present microcomputer discs. Optical holograms, produced by laser-beams, hold the promise of a desk top system having a capacity of one million million bits, enough to accommodate a good sized university library.

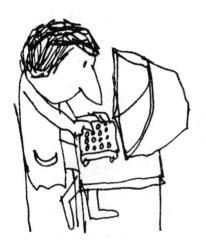

A similar revolution is upon us in the video world. The miniaturization of equipment and advanced capacities for speedy and accurate location of information on a video cassette or video disc provides the opportunity for producing interactive educational material previously limited to computers. It does not require too much imagination to think up several ways in which this facility could be of value and two of these have already been described. The essential problem to us as teachers is to know enough about these new technologies to allow us to utilize them and select those which have real value in helping us achieve our aims. We must not be seduced by the novelty nor must we let the opportunities they present pass us by.

EVALUATING TEACHING MATERIALS

Like all aspects of medical teaching the materials you produce, or intend to purchase, should be carefully evaluated. Forgive us for reminding you again that primary questions for audio and visual materials will always be 'Are they audible?' and 'Are they visible?'

A more detailed checklist of questions you should think through is provided in Figure 7.9.

FIGURE 7·9
EVALUATING TEACHING
MATERIALS (AFTER ROE
AND McDONALD)

Relevance of the material
- Why is it used?
- How does it relate to the course unit and other materials?

Content
- Is it factually correct?
- Is it balanced?
- Is it current?
- Does it make the right assumptions about students' prior knowledge?
- Is it pitched at the right level?

Structure
- Is it logical?
- Is it subdivided so that its structure is obvious?
- Is it an appropriate length?

Presentation
- Is the language clear?
- Are tables and illustrations used to best effect?
- Is the layout effective?
- Is it presented in an interesting fashion?
- If it is designed for independent study, can students use it without assistance?

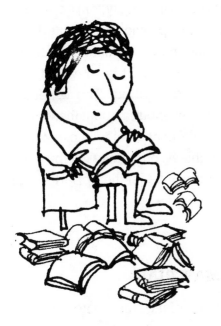

GUIDED READING

For a comprehensive guide to the wide range of teaching aids and their preparation, you will find considerable value in J. E. Kemp's *Planning and Producing Audio Visual Materials* (fourth edition), Harper and Rowe, New York, 1980. This book also provides a helpful theoretical and research base to the education aspects of using teaching aids.

Designing Instructional Text (Second Edition) by J. Hartley, Kogan Page, London, 1985.

Informed Professional Judgement: A Guide to Evaluation in Post-secondary Education, by E. Roe and R. McDonald, University of Queensland Press, Brisbane, 1983.

8: **HELPING STUDENTS LEARN**

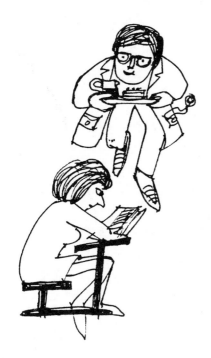

INTRODUCTION

The focus of this book so far has been on improving and broadening the range of teaching skills. Though we have assumed that the aim of doing so is for the ultimate benefit of the students, our emphasis has been on the personal development of the teacher. In this chapter we will introduce you to ideas which are not as widely represented in the teaching literature as those in other sections of the book. Nevertheless, we believe they have provided valuable new insights to us and to many of our colleagues. Thus, this chapter may appear to be more theoretical than previous ones but we include it without reservation because of the fundamental challenge it provides to the more traditional views of teaching.

Over the last few years a considerable body of evidence has accumulated which suggests that we need to become much more concerned with **how** our students learn. We need to appreciate that some of our students are having difficulties with their studies arising not just from lack of application or psychosocial problems, but from specific problems with the way they study and learn. We must also appreciate that some of these problems are directly attributable to the way we teach, organize courses and conduct assessments.

HOW STUDENTS LEARN

It seems that all students (and teachers) have distinctive **approaches to learning** which are influenced by many factors as shown in Figure 8.1.

FIGURE 8.1

A MODEL OF STUDENT

LEARNING

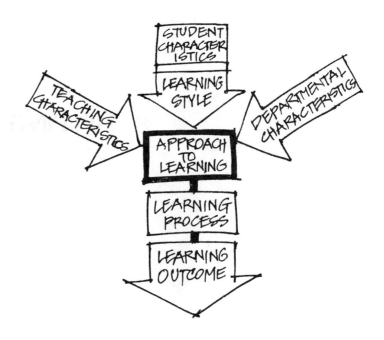

140

One of these factors is dependent on personality traits and is sometimes referred to as the preferred **learning style**. Other influences can be grouped under characteristics of the teaching and characteristics of the department organizing the course. In general, these two environmental influences seem to be more important than learning style in determining the students' approach to learning. The approach adopted subsequently determines the **learning process** or study method used by the student and this, in turn, affects the quality of the **learning outcome**.

Students can be observed to use one of three broad approaches to learning which can most conveniently be called surface, deep and strategic.

Students adopting a **surface approach** are predominantly motivated by a concern to complete the course or by a fear of failure. They intend to fulfil the assessment requirements of the course by memorizing factual material. The process they use to achieve this is rote learning. The outcome is, at best, a knowledge of factual information and a superficial level of understanding.

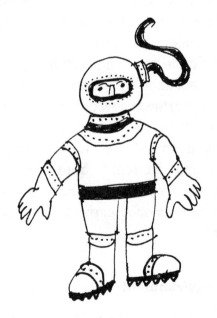

In contrast, students adopting a **deep approach** are motivated by an interest in the subject matter and by its vocational relevance. Their intention is to reach an understanding of the material. The process of achieving this varies between individual students and between students in different academic disciplines. The **operation learner** uses a process which relies on a logical step-by-step approach with a cautious acceptance of generalizations only when based on evidence. There is an attention to factual and procedural detail which may include rote learning. On the other hand, the **comprehension learner** uses a process in which the initial concern is for the broad outlines of the ideas with their inter-connections with previous knowledge. Such students make use of analogies and attempt to give the material personal meaning. However, the most effective process is that used by the so-called **versatile learner** in whom the outcome is a deep level of understanding based on a knowledge of broad principles supported by a sound factual basis. Versatile learning does not preclude the use of rote learning when the need arises, as it frequently does in science-based courses, but the students do so with a totally different intent from those using the surface approach.

Students demonstrating the **strategic approach** may be seen to use processes similar to both the deep and surface learner. The fundamental difference lies in their motivation and intention. Such students are motivated by the need to achieve high marks and to compete with others. The outcome is a variable level of understanding which depends on what is required by the course and the assessments.

The attributes we would hope for in a university student are very much those embodied in the deep approach. Disturbingly, the little evidence we have suggests that these attributes may not always be encouraged by teachers or achieved by students. Indeed there is some reason to believe that many of our teaching methods, curriculum structures and, particularly, our examining methods may be actively inhibiting the use of the deep approach and supporting the use of surface and strategic approaches.

LEARNING MORE EFFECTIVELY

The concepts outlined above are not only supported by a substantial body of evidence, but also match the impressions we have intuitively developed over many years of teaching students. We feel less comfortable proffering practical advice in the way we have done in previous chapters. This arises not only from the fact that we have only limited personal experience in applying these new concepts but also that very few other people have either! Even more importantly, there is only a limited amount of research demonstrating that changing students' approaches to learning can promote more effective learning outcomes. Nevertheless, we believe there is enough evidence to offer some general points of advice.

Improving the learning environment

This must be considered at various levels. At the broadest level is the educational philosophy underlying the whole medical school curriculum. There may be little you can do about this, but it might be as well to be aware that students from traditional medical schools seem to adopt the surface approach to a greater degree than students from problem-based schools.

142

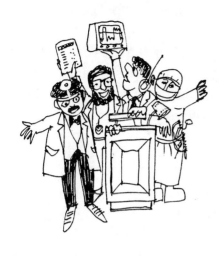

At another level, and one where you might be able to exert some influence, is the structuring of the curriculum. You should be aware that the fragmentation of the curriculum into a large number of courses taught by different specialists may be counterproductive to the development of deep approaches. The time available to each course is limited and so the opportunities for students to come to grips with the deeper implications and perspectives of subject matter are similarly restricted.

As most teachers reading this book will be working in a traditional school, it would seem to be important to introduce measures into courses which might encourage the use of the deep approach.

★ Ensure that the course objectives specify more than just facts and technical skills by giving suitable emphasis to higher level intellectual skills such as problem-solving, and to the exploration and development of attitudes.

★ Introduce teaching activities which require students to demonstrate a deep understanding of the subject matter or clinical problems. Do not allow students to 'get away' with only reproducing factual information.

★ Reduce the time allocated to didactic teaching to allow more time for group-based teaching and self-directed learning.

★ Decrease the amount of factual material that has to be memorized. Both time pressure and overloading with content are known to encourage the surface approach even in those intending to use the deep approach. These problems are prevalent in most medical schools.

★ Spend more contact time helping students understand and use basic principles. Get into the habit of expecting students to explain answers to questions. The frequent use of the word 'why' will quickly establish if the answer is based on memorization or on an understanding of an underlying principle.

★ **Most importantly**, review the assessment procedures. This is a critical task. If the assessment, course content and methods do not match the course objectives, then one could be the world's greatest teacher and make little impact on the students' learning. For example, an over-reliance on multiple-choice tests will almost certainly encourage the use of surface strategies. If you aim to have students understand the subject, then you must introduce forms of assessment which require them to demonstrate this understanding. This may mean the re-introduction of essays, project work, critical analysis of clinical problems and so on. Students should be fully informed about the content and methods, with examples provided.

Modifying teaching styles

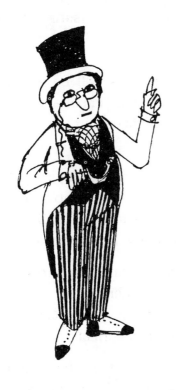

Teachers need to be aware that they have teaching style preferences for the same reasons that students have preferred learning styles. It is therefore unlikely that these preferences will match those of all students. The importance of this issue is uncertain but there is experimental evidence that a match of teaching and learning styles produces more effective learning.

It seems reasonable to suggest that teachers should develop skills which are likely to enhance the learning of all students, not just those with whom they may have a natural affinity. In the lecture situation, for instance, teachers who prefer to present material in a very logical and structured way may be popular with students with a preference for operation learning, but less so with students with a bent towards comprehension learning. The latter may be particularly assisted by the inclusion of an overview at the beginning of the lecture and analogies to set the material in context. In small groups, on the other hand, operation learners may be relatively uncomfortable in an unstructured situation.

As we know that operation learners are more prevalent in science-based disciplines, this may explain why lectures seem to dominate the teaching activities of most medical schools, often it seems with the collusion of both students and their teachers! Nevertheless, this may not be the ideal way of teaching important aspects of a medical course which might have more similarity to the social rather than physical sciences. It behoves you to appreciate this and to be prepared to broaden your approach in the best interest of the overall development and learning of your students.

Improving study skills

There seems little doubt that good study skills contribute to academic success, though in themselves they are not a guarantee of success. Skills must be tied to a positive attitude and motivation to the subject. Being well-organized and efficient in the use of time and resources is important. However, it is clear that there is no correct way to study, which may be why the use of study manuals and courses in study methods has not been very successful. Special counsellors may be valuable for students with very severe problems but there is a growing recognition that subject teachers should become more interested in helping students individually within the context of their own courses. An interview should make it possible to identify the problem area:

★ Social factors: too much time involved in extra-curricular activities; social motivation higher than academic.

★ Psychological factors: undue anxiety; interpersonal problems.

★ Specific study skill problems: poor scheduling of time; lack of study plan; inappropriate environment; inadequate preparation for examinations; poor examination techniques.

For further information and help with study skill counselling we refer you to the books by Main and by Gibbs which are recent enough to take into account some of the new understanding about student learning that we described earlier in the chapter.

GUIDED READING

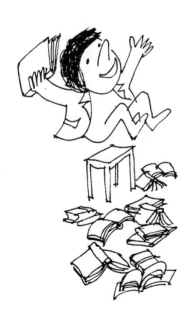

For a review of the research on which the ideas presented in this chapter have been based, we refer you to the following article:

Learning Styles and Approaches: Implications for Medical Education, by D.I. Newble and N.J. Entwistle, *Medical Education*, **20**, 1986, 162–175.

There are many books on study skills. Two that we find provide a balance of theory and practice and are not too cumbersome are A. Main's *Encouraging Effective Learning*, Scottish Academic Press, Edinburgh, 1980 and G. Gibbs' *Teaching Students to Learn: A Student-Centred Approach*, The Open University Press, Milton Keynes, 1981.

Another paperback book, containing a lot of detailed advice on both how to study and how to perform various academic tasks, is *A Guide to Learning Independently* by L. Marshall and F. Rowland, Longman Cheshire, Melbourne, 1981. Though written for students it is of equal value to teachers.

APPENDIX: WHERE TO FIND OUT MORE ABOUT MEDICAL EDUCATION

As a result of your involvement in teaching you may eventually wish to pursue in greater depth an interest in medical education. This section of the book will identify various resources which might be helpful.

BOOKS

We have already provided selected readings at the end of each chapter. There are some other texts which may be of more general interest and which cover a wider range than the selected readings.

Teaching and Learning in Medical School, Harvard University Press, 1961.
This book was written by a group of authors, headed by George Miller and Stephen Abrahamson, who subsequently became two of the most influential figures in the field of medical education. It is still one of the few comprehensive and comprehensible textbooks of medical education. Though now out of print, it is readily available in most medical school libraries.

The Medical Teacher (second edition), Churchill-Livingstone, Edinburgh, 1987. K. R. Cox and C. E. Ewan (eds.).
This recently revised book contains articles written by authors from all over the world, though with a majority of Australian contributions as the book developed from a popular series of articles which originally appeared in the Medical Journal of Australia. This book provides a useful resource for the teacher wishing to get a view of current issues in medical education. The articles are all brief and conclude with useful references and bibliography.

Teaching and Learning in Higher Education (fourth edition) R. M. Beard and J. Hartley, Harper and Row, London, 1984. This is an easy to read book dealing specifically with teaching at the tertiary level.

Problem-Based Learning: an Approach to Medical Education, Springer Publishing Co. Inc., New York, 1980.
This book, written by H. S. Barrows and R. M. Tamblyn, will be of interest to those concerned to introduce the problem-based approached into their teaching. Barrows has also produced another book entitled *How to Design a Problem Based Curriculum for the Preclinical Years*, Springer, 1985.

JOURNALS

Articles relating to medical education appear regularly in most of the major general medical journals. There are, however, several journals specifically concerned with publishing research and review articles in the field of medical education.

Medical Education

This is the official journal of the Association for the Study of Medical Education (ASME), which is the organization catering for individuals interested in medical education in the United Kingdom. It should be readily available in your medical school library.

The Association also produces an excellent series of booklets dealing with various aspects of medical education and has recently commenced a new series on medical education research. These are also published in the journal.

Journal of Medical Education

This is a publication of the Association of American Medical Colleges. As well as publishing articles relating to teaching, this journal also deals with the broader issues of the organization of medical education as it relates to the United States. It should also be readily available in your library.

Medical Teacher

This journal, formerly published by Update Publications is now produced by Carfax Publishing Company. It is not primarily a research journal. Rather, it is a journal containing review articles and descriptions of educational activities by medical teachers from around the world. It is an excellent source of ideas and information (address: Carfax Publishing Co. PO Box 25, Abingdon, Oxfordshire, OX14 3UE, UK).

Proceedings of the Research in Medical Education Conference

This is not strictly a journal, but is a very useful source of the most recent research in medical education, particularly that conducted in North America. It can be obtained from the Association of American Medical Colleges (see under 'Organizations').

Many other journals carry articles relating to higher education and sometimes specifically to medical education. Rather than trying to produce a comprehensive list we would suggest using the references of appropriate articles appearing in the medical educational journals as the way of identifying additional journals likely to be of interest.

OTHER RESOURCES

BLAT Centre for Health and Medical Education

This British organization produces a small and inexpensive publication called *Information*. It provides a news section giving details of such things as conferences and courses. It also contains research abstracts and book reviews. Other sections deal with descriptions and reviews of teaching and learning materials and information about new educational equipment (address: BMA House, Tavistock Square, London, WC1H 9JP).

World Health Organization

The WHO has been very active for many years in the field of medical education. It frequently commissions experts to write review documents. A list of such publications might be available in your library. If not, you could contact your regional WHO office or write direct to Distribution and Sales, 1211 Geneva 27, Switzerland.

The following are some examples of WHO publications which may be of interest:

Educational Strategies for the Health Professions, G. E. Miller and T. Fülöp (eds.), Public Health Paper No. 52, 1973.
Competency Based Curriculum Development in Medical Education, W. C. McGaghie, G. E. Miller, A. W. Sajid, T. V. Telder, Public Health Paper No. 68, 1978.
Personnel for Health Care, Case Studies of Educational Programmes, F. M. Katz and T. Fülöp (eds.), Public Health Paper Nos. 70, 1978 and 71, 1980.
Assessing Health Workers' Performance, F. M. Katz, and R. Snow, Public Health Paper, No. 72, 1980.
Educational Handbook for Health Personnel, WHO Offset Publication No. 35, Geneva, 1981.
Community-Based Education for Health Personnel, Technical Report Series, WHO, 1986.

TRAINING OPPORTUNITIES

Many tertiary institutions have individuals or units whose job is to provide assistance to teachers. We would strongly recommend you make full use of these resources. Alternatively, you could elect to attend courses run by other organizations in your area or even overseas. The WHO supports regional teacher training centres which offer short courses for medical teachers and even degree courses in health personnel education.

Some universities and departments of medical education also run courses of various types and some have well developed fellowship programmes for local and overseas postgraduate students. Well known examples of such institutions include the Division of Research in Medical Education at the University of Southern California in Los Angeles, the Center for Educational Development at the University of Illinois College of Medicine in Chicago and the Centre for Medical Education at the University of Dundee.

OVERSEAS TRAVEL

Generally speaking, people concerned with medical education are a friendly and helpful lot. Should you be travelling, do not hesitate to write to any individual or institution you may wish to visit and observe at first hand educational activities or facilities which have interested you during your reading. If you come from a traditional medical school, you should attempt to visit one of the less conventional schools such as McMaster University in Hamilton, Canada; Limberg University in Maastricht, The Netherlands; Ben Gurion University of the Negev, Beer-Sheva, Israel; or Newcastle University, Australia. Other institutions which are currently experimenting with alternative curricula include Southern Illinois University and the University of New Mexico.

ORGANIZATIONS

As your interest in medical education grows you may wish to join an association of like minds or attend one of the national or international conferences which are held each year. The following is a list of some of the most well known English speaking organizations which conduct major annual conferences.

Association for Medical Education in Europe (AMEE)

This is an umbrella organization for national medical educational associations in Europe. It is also well supported by the WHO. In addition it provides a regular forum for the meeting of medical school deans from Europe and sometimes from other parts of the world.

Further information can be obtained from the Secretary, c/o The Medical School, University of Edinburgh, Teviot Place, Edinburgh EH8 9AG, Scotland.

Association for the Study of Medical Education (ASME)

This is also a European organization with a largely British membership but with a significant number of members from other countries. It caters for individuals with an interest in medical education and provides a forum for communication of ideas and information. It organizes conferences and workshops and produces several publications including the well known journal, Medical Education.

Further details can be obtained from the Secretary, Centre for Medical Education, University of Dundee, 2, Roseangle, Dundee, DD1 4LR, Scotland.

Association of American Medical Colleges

This is another umbrella organization covering medical schools in America. It holds an annual meeting and in conjunction with this is held the Research in Medical Education Conference. This meeting provides the major annual gathering of workers in the field of medical education in the United States and Canada.

Further information can be obtained from the AAMC, One Dupont Circle NW, Washington, D.C. 20036.

Australasian and New Zealand Association for Medical Education

This association is comparable with ASME. It holds an annual conference and also supports state and regional groups which meet on a regular basis. It publishes a Bulletin several times a year.

Further information can be obtained from the Secretary, C/- Centre for Medical Education, Research and Development, University of New South Wales, P.O. Box 1, Kensington, NSW, 2033, Australia.

INDEX